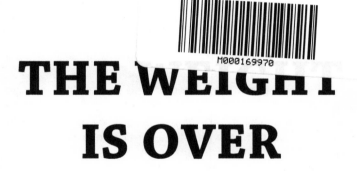

THE WEIGHT
IS OVER

My Journey to Loving My Body
From the Outside In

Syleena Johnson

Strategic Book Publishing and Rights Co.

Strategic Book Publishing and Rights Co., LLC
USA | Singapore
www.sbpra.com

For information about special discounts for bulk purchases, please contact Strategic Book Publishing and Rights Co., LLC. Special Sales, at bookorder@sbpra.net.

ISBN: 978-1-948858-06-9

Co-writer: Amera McCoy

Book Cover Design: Javon Fairley, JV Grafix and Jamilah A. Mason, A Work of Jam

Book synopsis: Shari Nycole Welton

Photography: O.Jay Rice Photography

Hair: LaToya Alexander

Makeup: Christian Balenciaga

Styling: Zoe Dupree

Dedication

To my husband, Kiwane Garris, and my two baby boys, KJ and Kingston. Because you gave me the stories, the strength, and the space to create. I love you.

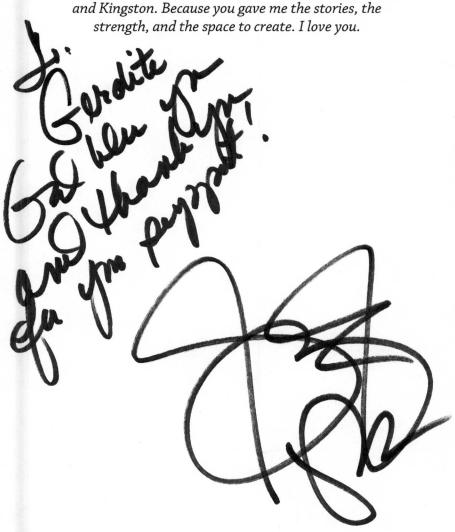

Table of Contents

FOREWORD

by Michael Dyson

Weight Time

I can still remember the first time I heard Syleena's voice. I was living in Chicago, sampling its urban wonders and taking in its cultural splendors. Among them was the vibrant music scene the city was known for, especially its blues rhythms and its soul music fare. As a native Detroiter, I was a harshly competitive judge. My ears had been shaped by the piercing and poignant stylings of the Queen of Soul, Aretha Franklin, whose vocal majesty set the standard of great performance for the nation. Not to mention the thrilling harmonies of the Temptations and the Four Tops, and the sweet melodies of The Supremes. So I knew music; I couldn't be hoodwinked by the latest fad or bamboozled by a would-be diva who was really a low-rent vocal fake. Marvin Gaye and Tami Terrell made sure I knew the real thing when I heard it.

So, with a bit of a lyrical chip on my shoulder, and with my musical snobbery at full tilt, you can imagine my utter surprise when I was blown away by a sonic tornado that swept me into its wake in 2001 when my car radio, to switch metaphors, unleashed Syleena's volcanic fury on "I Am Your Woman." What a revelation it was. Her smoky vocals bathed in an edifying rasp. Her voice dripped in sweet vibrato that ranged from a downhome guttural growl formed in a plangent contralto that effortlessly swooped up to a soaring soprano in forceful falsetto. All I wanted to know was who is the woman behind that voice? What is her story, the pain and suffering that clearly went into making that voice howl in controlled agony, all of the anecdotes of joy and triumph, the grace notes of struggle and salvation that might be heard even more clearly if I, if we, could have a conversation with her?

Well, the wait is over. Or as Syleena reminds us, the weight is over. And she gives it to us swift and honest, rugged, rough and real. The ups and downs, the highs and lows, the successes and failures, narrated with the persistent drumbeat of resurrection and redemption playing beneath it all. This is not a typical rags-to-riches tale, though there are plenty of gladrags and enormous riches, not just of pocket, but of person, of spirit, of heart and soul. Syleena tells it all here, stories of a childhood full of love and food, but also a time that sowed the seeds of self-doubt and overeating, later blossoming in eating to console loneliness, eating to compensate for spiritual emptiness.

But there are hungers that go deeper than the belly, and Syleena touches on them: hunger for intimacy more than sex, hunger for fulfillment more than material rewards, hunger for joy beyond the thrill of chart success. She is brutally honest, too, about her self-image as a tall, statuesque woman who towers over so many men and women. She paid a price for her stature, and she lets all of us in on the relentless self-doubt that comes from being an Amazon before Jeff Bezos became the world's richest man by branding the term. She shares her struggle with weight, with how she should look in an entertainment world obsessed with size and appearance.

Syleena writes insightfully about her body, as an athlete who was good at tennis, basketball and track, as a black woman forced to address colorism and skin shade and hair texture, and everything, all the trials and tribulations, the tests of will, and endurance, that come with being black and female in America. She addresses the weight of being a wife and mother, of meeting expectations of others and herself as she battles childhood health traumas for her son and the emotional and psychological weight that gloms on to the psyches of conscientious and industrious women.

Syleena leaves no stone unturned: her nearly lifelong quest to right the scales of her own self-perception, self-consciousness, and self-reconstruction, as she gains expertise in nutrition and diet in the effort to make her body and soul conform to a higher calling, and a greater measure of her worth than the affirmation of a superfluous society, or on scales that record her weight. She talks about being a woman, a girlfriend, a friend, a mate, a partner, a soldier in the war to grow into her best self, her most morally and physically beautiful self, while fighting the corrosive, and corrupting, weight of depression, judgmentalism and unrealistic expectations. It's all here, and a lot more besides.

After nearly twenty years of enjoying her musical genius, of sampling her extraordinary voice, I have learned that Syleena is a fierce and formidable sprit whose inner beauty is even more impressive than her external beauty. I have learned that her height as a striking model of exemplary womanhood is matched by the heights, and depths, she has scaled to become the woman she is today. I am so glad, and you will be too, that the weight is finally over, and the story of the woman behind the voice I heard all those years ago is even more amazing than I thought. Don't take my word. Read it for yourself.

PREFACE

It's 4 a.m., and today is the day I will run 13.1 miles straight, with no chaser. Four months of training for this race. Four months of sweating, praying, dieting, strength training, and praying some more. But, is it enough? Will it be enough? Oh God, my girlfriends Charita and Eddy are right next to me with a glorious look of hope and optimism in their eyes as they cheer me on every fifteen minutes.

"You're going to do it, Syleena. We are so proud of you, girl," they say as they slip on their sneakers with ease. Perhaps they know that, for them, it's just another race and another medal to hang with the rest of the many they have already achieved over the years.

At forty-two and forty-eight years old, they have accomplished marathon after marathon and even triathlons. But, do they know that on the inside I am terrified of what is to come? Do they know I just wrapped up shooting a movie, have been traveling in and out, and I am in the middle of working my sixth studio *Chapter* album?

My Hal Higdon half marathon training log was designed to prepare me for this day, but I must say that I haven't followed it to a T. So, today on that starting line it's going to be me, Eddy, Charita, and Jesus! *I hope my legs don't fall off* is all that is repeating in my head as I join the girls in my kitchen to make my prerun energy drink. Now we are in the truck on our way to the race. It's 5 a.m., we need to be there no later than 6:45, and it's an hour away.

Deep breathing as I fidget with my iPod, making sure the battery is charged and is working fine and dandy. My iPod had been shutting off in the middle of my runs during my training, and Lord knows I don't have time for that. I cannot run without music, so when the music stops, I will too, and we can't have that either. I didn't do all this work and drive all the way out to Peachtree City, Georgia, to walk. So this iPod is going to have to get it together. And if it cuts off, I am prepared to write a scathing letter to Apple.

Finally, we have arrived. Even though the sun has not yet risen to reveal the pink-ruffled skirts and neon-yellow socks that seem to be the run-like-a-diva uniform, I can still see a swarm of women of all shapes, ages, and sizes lined up to catch the shuttle that will take us to the starting line for what will probably become either the hardest or the easiest race of our lives. Every woman is different, and I am sure there are some seasoned runners out there like Charita and Eddy. I know it will definitely be the hardest for me! I have run ten miles, but I didn't get around to that additional three, and right now in my mind I don't know how to quiet my thoughts to prepare myself for this race. So, I will just smile and nod in agreement.

"Yep, I am going to turn up, ladies" is what my mouth says, but my mind is shaking its head, saying, *Chile, what have you gotten yourself into this time?*

We walk up to the shuttle line and three lovely black women say to me, "Hey, you are Syleena Johnson from *R&B Divas.* Can we take a picture with you?"

"Absolutely," I reply, no makeup and all, looking like a hot mess.

Then, suddenly, one of them says, "You always about that fitness, girl."

Then something inside of me clicks. Women recognize that I am fighting for optimal health. They see what I am doing, and they appreciate it. This race will be an inspiration to others, and so the fear in me starts to slowly seep away and transform into pride. I began to poke my chest out a bit mentally. I then replied, "Thank you, and yes, I am. You ladies have a great race." Suddenly I became Syleena Johnson, SheLean Lifestyle Health & Fitness CEO and President, and it felt good.

While waiting in line for the bathroom, I still have butterflies. Even though my mind is ready, my body is trying not to hear it. However, a bathroom break may release some unnecessary rumblings in my tummy. I just hope they don't call my wave while I'm sitting on the toilet. Oh Lord, help me, I am so nervous. Jesus, be a way to make this line go faster! It's 7:15 a.m. The 5K runners are being summoned to the starting line. Oh boy, the 13.1 mile half marathon is next, at 7:30 a.m., and finally I am about to use the restroom. Thank God, because running while having to pee would simply not work for my goal of running nonstop. As I walk out of the restroom, I see Charita and Eddy waiting for me as they stretch their legs in preparation for the race. My husband, Kiwane, and family friend Reggie stand by with a video camera and some hand sanitizer.

"Wave one," I hear screamed through a bullhorn. Oh crap, that's us! We rush over, scanning the thousands of runners as we inch our way up to the starting line. Wave one is gone! That was our wave! Did we miss it? Oh God! Wave two is announced over the bullhorn. Well, I guess we can just slip into this wave. The wave you are in is determined by the time you run. I registered at a ten-minute mile, but in actuality I just want to finish. I probably should've entered into wave five, just to be safe. Oh wait, there is no wave five. I anticipate my average running pace to be a minute longer than it was in my training, but when the starter said go, the momentum had me fired up inside. *Maybe I'll run like a Kenyan*, I thought. Now I'm just waiting.

Looking at Kiwane, smiling for the camera, laughing with Charita and Eddy about this journey that is about to take place, I'm ignoring the butterflies and urging them to pinch me so that I can wake up from this surreal dream. It's time.

"Two minutes to takeoff," yells that annoying announcer. Palms are sweaty, mind is racing, sun is rising, and the countdown starts. I lower my shades over my eyes, cue the music on my iPod: "Five, four, three, two, one—GO!"

The Daughter

"Brenda's Got a Baby" – Tupac

Everyone who knows me knows my mother, Brenda Thompson. She is the center of the family and has always been prevalent in my life. Looking back on my childhood, I can recount the lessons in body image, nutrition, and beauty taught by my mother. I can say there were not many, for many reasons. Body image, weight management, nutrition, and beauty were not popular topics in my home, or in the home of the average African-American family, for that matter.

My mom and her sisters were considered the "Pretty Girls" when they were in high school. What I mean by pretty is fair-skinned with long, silky hair. You know, the stereotypical ideal of what society feels is beautiful. Ironically, though, in my mother's day, having fair skin and long, silky hair as a black woman was a double-edged sword. You were pretty by society's standards, but in the black community you were a half-breed, a redbone, or a wannabe white woman. It's a broad concept, but I say it with love. The black community has been known to praise each other based on skin color. We, like those who judge us, view fair skin as beautiful. Though times are changing and things are not as bad, it is still a stigma many generations have dealt with in the past, and, unfortunately, in the present.

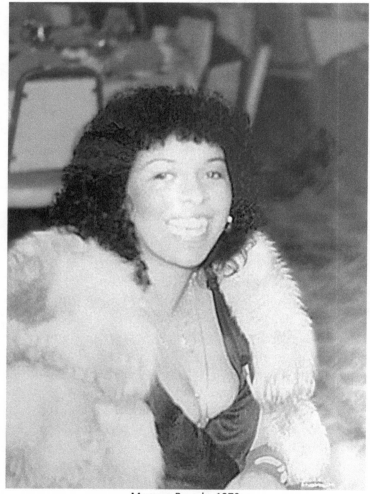

Momma Brenda, 1970

My mom kept herself in fairly good shape as best as she could, even though she smoked cigarettes and drank alcohol. Most of her post-baby bounce back was due to her amazing genetics.

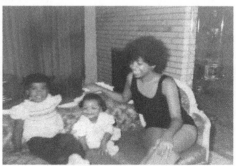

Sylette, Syleecia, and Mom 1974

I can remember her, my aunts, and my grandmother dressing up in leotards and working out in the basement. As a young child, I was right next to my mom and sisters exercising to Jane Fonda and Denise Austin workout tapes. I guess this is where I was first introduced to physical fitness as a brand, not knowing that this would be imbedded in my future forever. Doing workout videos was nothing more than just the thing we did occasionally with the women in my family. I never really assessed the purpose for it during that time. Looking back on it now, I know the exercises they did in the basement were meaningful to her in some way.

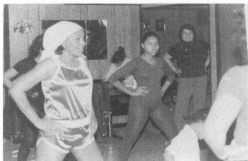

Me at 5 years old exercising in the basement with aunts, grandma, and mom.

3

Whether it was her way of staying in shape, keeping up with the latest trends, or just a healthy way of spending time with family, even back then there were remnants of body image. Maybe she just wanted to look her best, only then it didn't mean as much as it does today.

Even though my mom could be boogie or critical of others, when it came to my sisters and me, my mother tried to be as positive as she could. She constantly told us we were beautiful, and, given our active lifestyles, we were far from overweight or even thinking about weight as an issue. My mother did think I was very tall for a girl, but that didn't impact my views on body image negatively. Actually, for the most part she was right. I was a tall young lady standing at five ten by the age of twelve, but my height would be an advantage later on in life as I entered into the world of sports.

As a child, we lived on a soul food diet and could eat heavily without gaining a pound. In fact, we were encouraged to clean our plates. This was the mantra of most black families, and I suspect there is a percentage that still receives that encouragement to this day. My mother, along with the rest of the family, viewed food as a way of showing love. Our meals, though unhealthy, represented family and fulfillment, and we didn't worry much about what role food played in our overall health. I enjoyed our family dinners and the food we shared. There weren't any instances where I even thought of food or the behavior of the family's thoughts toward food as negative.

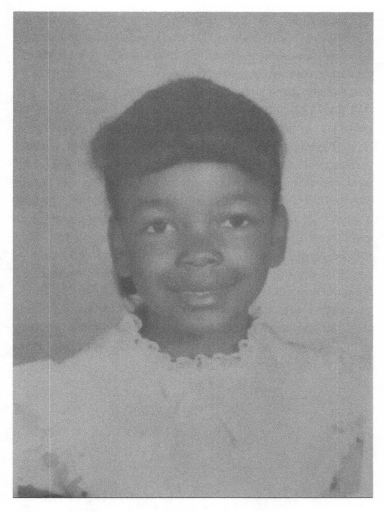

4th grade

As I got older and learned more about my own behavior and thoughts toward food, I realized that how we choose and consume food is closely related to how we were taught to eat as children. Consequently, if I love food and eat all day, I could genuinely believe that I was loving myself. I would later find out how wrong I was.

5

As a child I can't remember any negative connotation toward the food we ate or the image our family had around outward appearance. However, I do vaguely remember my mom mentioning intermittently, "You know, even though you can eat three cheeseburgers now and not gain a pound, that doesn't mean that it won't catch up with you when you get older, young lady." Boy, was she right. Since I was athletic, I never really gained much weight. However, I do remember through the midst of everything my dad always cooked his own food. He was always conscious of what he was eating. Maybe he knew something I didn't at the time, but, again, as a child you are not often thinking of eating meals separate from your family's standard dinner. Therefore, my dad's independent eating behaviors were of no concern to any of us, but I am my father's child. I was intrigued by this and frequently would eat from his interesting menu of salmon croquettes and vegetable medleys that he would name zucchini. He would also drink an assortment of hot teas, which I now know as a singer was actually very important for his voice and overall well-being.

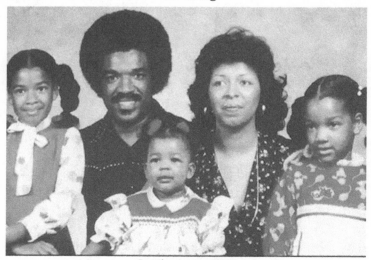

Family picture 1978

Ideally, my relationship with my body was positive. I was fit in more ways than one: first, I "fit" my mother's image, and second, I was physically fit for all three of the sports that I participated in from elementary school all the way up to college.

My perception of body image was nonexistent until things outside of my homelife began to put a spotlight on it. There is one memory that sticks with me from childhood, because it was my introduction to body image and/or awareness of others' opinions of someone else's body. My mother took my sister to the doctor, and commentary from the physician suggested my sister was overweight or in need of losing weight. My mother told the entire family about the comments from the doctor, and my sister was teased about the situation by my cousins and other family members. At the time, I didn't know any better, so I teased her as well. It was unheard of for anyone in my family to have a weight issue. Not only was it unheard of, but the idea that a doctor would give such information out without advising how to mentally handle this situation added insult to injury. I guess, because he was a family physician, he wasn't really concerned with what this may have done to a child. But, then again, black people aren't really concerned with getting therapy anyway, so I suppose that was irrelevant at the time. Today, I look back and know that situation had to be extremely uncomfortable for my mom and for my sister.

I would say my sister was chubby in the face, but far from overweight. The way my family dealt with the issue of her weight was the first negative seed that was planted in my subconscious. Though I think of all the ways I could have handled this better myself, I was eight years old at the time and wouldn't have known better. My mother, on the other hand, set the example and wasn't very encouraging to my sister either. In my family, when there was an issue, it was either swept under the rug or the person with the issue was forced to deal with it and get over it. Either way was unproductive. This is where therapy or, at the very least, positive encouragement could have changed the entire outcome of this story.

With little girls, some topics are very fragile and should be handled with care, especially if you want them to grow to be somewhat stable women. I have to believe that my mom did the best she could with what she knew. If you yourself weren't handled with care growing up, then I guess you can't handle others with care either. It was around this time that I picked up on a number of body image issues that were subconscious seeds for me. The issue regarding body image was not directed specifically at me nor did it involve me. I was merely a bystander learning the good and bad habits that our society creates. It suddenly didn't matter that I had a loving family and positive relationships at home; every encounter began to plant a seed and create a view on body image that I wasn't ready to accept.

Around the age of twelve I hit puberty and began to suffer from acne. The teasing I experienced in school was extreme; students would call me names like "pizza face" and other horrible acne names. This experience did a number on my self-esteem and planted seeds of insecurity related to my face. I carried these insecurities around with me everywhere I went. It was a very difficult time for me, and I believe it was the start of a wave of deep low self-esteem. The main issue back then was that I suffered through acne when I probably didn't have to. My mom didn't take me to a dermatologist, not because she didn't want to, but because she didn't know to. I am sure she was just as distraught with my face breaking out as I was, but she just didn't know what to do. All she knew to say was, "Stop eating all that candy,"

"It's the sugar," or, "You're not drinking enough water." Ironically, once again she was right.

However, while those little things do aggravate inflammation and perpetuate bacteria in the body by breaking down the immune system, acne is a disorder that oftentimes calls for medicinal treatment. Adolescent acne is prone to happen, and some have it worse than others, but the phase is a common step for many young people. Unfortunately, I would grow to have acne way into adulthood. Of course, my mom loved me through it, but the resources and specialists available today seemed out of reach for me as a child.

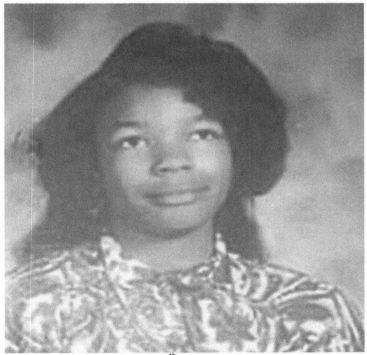

7th grade

It wasn't until I reached college that I found a dermatologist in Chicago who would change my life. Turns out I have sensitive skin, like millions of other people in the world, and I still break out today if exposed to certain foods, stress, hormonal fluctuations, and dirty makeup brushes. I now know what to avoid to maintain reasonably clear skin. Although I know these simple solutions now, the trials and errors I experienced as a child were traumatizing to me, and some of those negative feelings resurface when I meet new people. It's my face. It's the first thing a person sees when they meet you, and whether or not people admit it, they judge how they will treat you from there. It takes a special person to be able to ignore comments of others and love yourself anyway. These times probably caused the disconnection from loving what I saw on the outside to connect with what was great about me on the inside. I can fully understand how some kids retract from society and fold into a shell, never really emerging to be themselves.

Kids can be brutal toward other kids, and the impacts can last a lifetime if there is not enough blatant love to combat it. As for me, I moved through my acne phase with these seeds buried in the soil of my soul, just waiting to be watered and to bloom as an adult.

Despite my acne, many good years and good things ensued as well, including the fact that I was praised for my body. Between the ages of fourteen and seventeen I pretty much settled in height and filled out into a woman. I was five ten and 155 pounds, and instead of looking like one of the students, I looked more like one of the teachers. I was taller than the average girl and, in most cases, the average boy as well. I was in shape, so I didn't have negative feelings about my body. In fact, my confidence started to build as I was considered to be one of the more "good-looking" girls in school. Even though this may have been the case, I didn't always feel that way. I always thought others were prettier, and once I hit high school the beginning stages of seeds from my past started to grow.

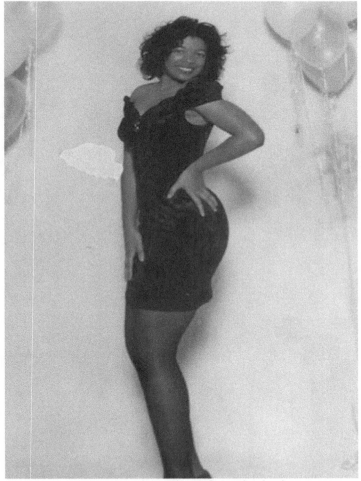

Sophomore dance Thornridge High School

The Athlete

"Ballin" – Jim Jones

High school was somewhat of a roller coaster for me. It was filled with good memories, from prom queen, to state finals, to bad memories, like fighting in the school library and making a whole lot of bad choices. It is around this time you begin to test your limits mentally and physically. I realized my physical composition was a bit more developed than my peers. Everything about me physically was exaggerated in high school because I was more developed than the majority of students my age. Honestly, I reveled in the attention and enjoyed it, even when it became something that would get me sent to the dean's office on a consistent basis.

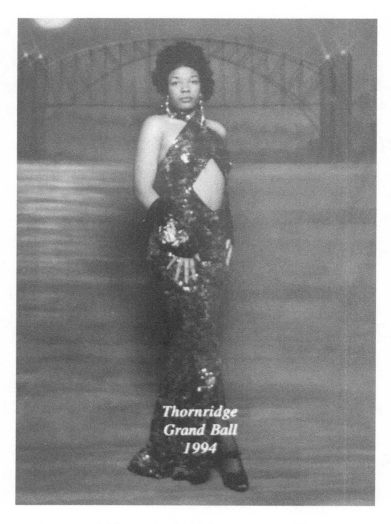

*Thornridge
Grand Ball
1994*

It seemed like everything I wore was offensive, and teachers would send me to the office. Pants too tight? Go to the office. Skirt two inches above the knee? Go to the office. Dress too fitted? Go to the office. It got so bad that I started to question what I should wear to school. To make matters worse, my mom would call me into her bedroom every morning before I went to school to do a full inspection of my outfit. It was annoying at first, but then it just became routine. Imagine that the first communication between you and your maternal mirror is criticism. Interesting the things you can get used to. Perhaps God was preparing me for the music business.

But then something cool happened. I met a crew of girls from choir that literally stood anywhere from five nine to five eleven and were just as filled out as I was. One joined the tennis team with me, and her father was a retired NBA/overseas basketball player. The others were just tall, I guess, but they were as pretty as they were tall and shared the same talents as I did musically. Moreover, I wasn't the tallest girl on the basketball team anymore. There was a girl that stood six four who was new to the team. I was actually able to move into the small forward/shooting guard position because she was clearly the perfect candidate for center. I wasn't the biggest girl in the group anymore, and this was a huge boost to my self-esteem. It was also really cool to know that I was not alone and was, in fact, normal. I began to realize that different was acceptable. I suppose it is all about how you choose to view things.

Well, according to my coaches, I was the perfect height, weight, and size for every sport that I participated in. They even bragged about how I would be great for college basketball. Unbeknownst to them, that was a dream of mine, and I had intended to work hard enough to do just that. However, as you can see, God had a different plan for me altogether.

For those of you who don't know my first love is sports, I am an athlete through and through. As a matter of fact, I was a three-sport athlete, participating in tennis, basketball, and track. I am competitive, and as an active athlete I was confident. It's important to know the body image I carried of myself in high school, because it was untainted, for the most part. In my mind, there was nothing that I could not do physically. I've always been tall, but my height was less and less of an issue and more and more of an advantage. I quickly became popular in high school for my athletic stature. All the while, being as active as I was, I could eat terribly, gain no weight, and see no difference in my body at all.

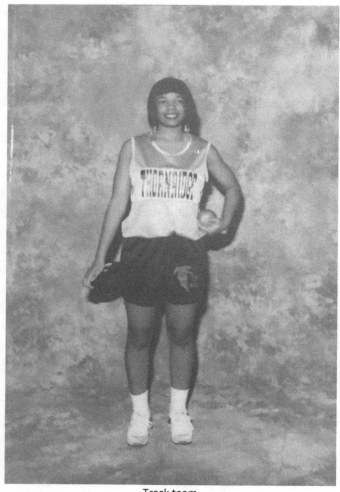

Track team

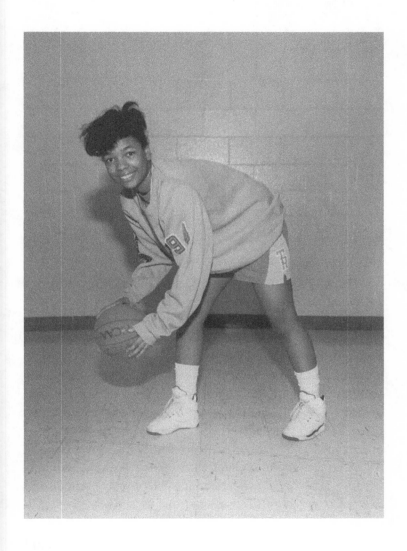

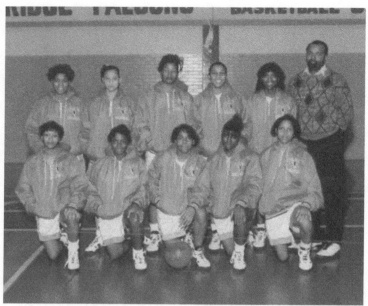

Thornridge High School Sophomore Girls Basketball Team (top center)

My body remained beautiful and celebrated by my peers. I was the perfect size for sports, and so I *never* thought of myself as fat or overweight. I actually thought my body was fabulous. The only time I can recall being insecure was during a cheerleading tryout. Like many schools, cheerleaders were the popular pretty girls who dated the athletes. Though I was considered to be both popular and pretty, I was not a cheerleader. I was the polar opposite, being the girl who played the sports with the guys every opportunity that presented itself. Not being viewed as the prissy stereotype of a cheerleader didn't bother me much, because I had been a cheerleader in elementary school, and it wasn't anywhere near as vigorous as actually playing in the game.

The thrill of the game was much more attractive, and I didn't care if I had to have skinned knees and sprained ankles to participate. My basketball coach said we had to be in a sport during off-season to stay in shape year-round, Myself a few other girls from the team thought we'd be slick and do something easy. Besides, it was football season, and to us cheerleading was basically a reason to dress up and scream while you got front row seats to view young men in tight pants. Seemed like a foolproof plan—until those tryouts came.

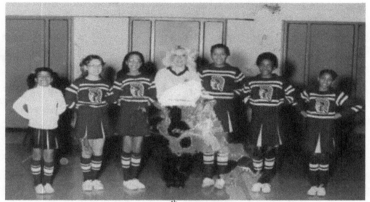

St. John the Baptist 7th grade cheerleading team
(Pictured 1st from the left)

When we found out that we had to do flips and splits and fit into suits the size of a baby doll, things quickly came into perspective. This cheerleading crap is harder than what I remember! Chile, when it became my turn to do a round-off flip, I immediately went into what seemed to be the loudest flip in the flip history books. I tell you, when I mounted, the floor had to shake, if not the entire building. Five feet ten inches and 155 pounds of muscle, fat, water, and bones soaring through the air at rapid speed just to get folks to clap for somebody else? After that landing it became clear that this was not the plan.

I remember the snickering and laughing of the already stick-thin and featherweight cheerleaders along with their evil leader, the captain. I just wanted to find their spirit stick and throw it, hitting them upside the head with it. I couldn't really blame them, though. I was a hot mess. But dang, couldn't they have waited until they got home to laugh? The rest of my teammates also failed miserably. So some of us went out for the cross-country team, while others, like myself, reported to the tennis courts. The tennis coach was my English honors teacher, so I thought maybe that wouldn't be too bad either. Wrong again, but it was so much fun that I didn't care. One of my Amazon best girlfriends I mentioned earlier was on the team with me. I enjoyed watching her throw her racket at her opponent every time she started losing. It was a blast! Eventually, I actually got pretty good at tennis and became first doubles. And, as an added bonus, I created lasting friendships through laughter and competition. I still keep in touch with some of my tennis teammates to this day, and we still laugh at old tennis stories. So, it was meant to be.

However, even though that entire cheerleading debacle was quite hilarious and one for the books, deep down inside it subconsciously watered one of those seeds inside of me I spoke of earlier. I began to wonder if my fantastic size was too much for the real world that says a woman should be smaller than a man. Would my size prevent me from being girlfriend material? It was the only time I could remember feeling insecure about my size in high school. I was larger in stature than all of the current cheerleaders, so they probably weren't going to choose me anyway. Either way, I am still competitive, so in my eyes nothing beats a failure but a try. Plus, those front row seats to blooming male body parts in tights wasn't exactly a bad incentive.

I also learned a valuable lesson: you can never judge a book by its cover. I learned that cheerleaders are athletes too. It really doesn't matter what sport I was in, I was always

going to be a team player, so, \
tennis, I had planned to do my best
of feeling inadequate from not mak
rug. This was just what I was taught t
moving, with the attitude that some
for some than others. Deep down insid
feel like the real reason why I didn't ma
team was because I was too big. Feelings   teem
once lost were now found again, and thos seeds began to
grow. Nonetheless, I would go on to finish high school as a
three-sport athlete, with a 3.2 grade point average, and a
prom queen title. In those moments in my life, I can honestly
say that I truly felt accomplished and beautiful with no
pressure. I never would have thought that it would be a
long time coming before I felt that way again.

Along came my glorious college years. I managed to
stay fairly fit through the summer and held onto my athletic
physique and the confidence that came along with it—until
I entered my freshman year. I fell victim to the "freshman
fifteen," gaining fifteen pounds before I could say White
Castle cheeseburger. I went from 165 to a smooth 180! I
think I was shocked that my body began to gain weight from
my bad eating habits. Previously, this was never an issue for
me. Usually during the summer, I would be in basketball
camps staying pretty active. Unfortunately, I cut my ties
with basketball in my senior year, so my activities decreased.

My coach was not the most encouraging when it came
to me continuing in the sport after my back injury. I felt like
he gave up on me. He treated me like I had just started
playing basketball that week, when he had been coaching
me since the seventh grade. I suppose my fear of
experiencing pain didn't make it any better, but I just knew
that he would encourage me through this, based on our
player-coach bond. Guess I was wrong, because every time I

ot on the court, I was afraid that my back would
, and that it could be permanent. Strangely, I felt like I
uldn't confide in him. It was an inflamed sciatic nerve due
to improper shock absorption in my tennis shoes. Actually,
some stretching and patience would have been enough to
get me through. But when you aren't really interested in a
player's development and success, you're really not
interested in teaching them how to prevail through tough
times either.

Maybe I needed too much from him because of my
father's absence when it came to my involvement in sports.
During this time, the only game my father ever went to for
any of my sports was senior parent night for basketball.
Keep in mind, I played three sports. My basketball coach
picked me up and dropped me off from seventh grade until
I walked away from the sport altogether my senior year.
However, I began to see him differently. Consequently, this
caused us to argue quite a bit and eventually tarnish my
love for playing the game.

I ended up choosing to go downstate with my speech
team for group interpretation instead of participating in my
basketball team's sectional tournament. They ended up
losing, and my group interpretation team won. Now, I don't
know if they lost because I wasn't there, but I just know that
I won because I wasn't. Either way, I walked away from
basketball, which left me inactive. So, when I got to college I
opened myself up to new ideas of getting in shape.

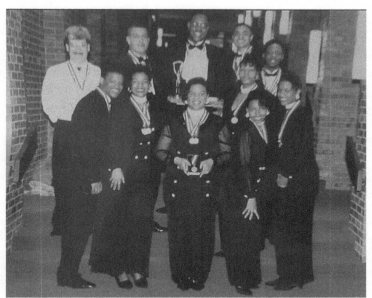

Thornridge High School Dramatic Interpretation Team
(I'm pictured 2nd from the left in the bottom row. Top row 4th is
Francois Battiste and next to him is the late Nelsan Ellis.)

My first college roommate, a pharmacy major and fitness fanatic, was in her junior year. Her drive and love for fitness began to encourage me to explore new aspects of health and fitness. She was, and still is, a vegetarian and was pretty much eating clean at the young age of twenty. I didn't start eating clean or even understand the importance of that until I was twenty-eight, so, to me, she was ahead of her time. I started doing aerobics with her, then I started taking some classes, and not long after began teaching classes of my own. My obsession with fitness took on a life of its own while I was in college. I even started playing intramural basketball. I was again in familiar territory. I was still in shape throughout, but I can recall times when body image and expectations began to interrupt my routine thoughts of self.

I remember my second college roommate was struggling with body image. Ironically, she was a beautiful dark-skinned girl with an amazing body. She was extremely fit and had a wonderful personality, but she was quite insecure due to her skin color. I remember how she used to worship another girl on the track team that was light-skinned, five nine, with long, brown, kinky curly hair. A "Mixed Chick" I presumed. She was indeed very beautiful, stunning even, and most of the men on campus, especially the male athletes, salivated every time she walked by.

Drake University was known for its track team. It hosted the famous Drake Relays that brought teams from all across America to compete every year. So, being on the track team was a big deal at this university. As a result, those on the track team were looked at as celebrities. They were special, and this girl clearly seemed to be that and more. Personally, I thought my roommate was just as beautiful, but I understood the stereotypical bubble that we all lived in. I understood that this girl would get more things offered to her in life, be paid more attention to, and pretty much have her pick of the litter throughout her life when it came to men. I'd seen this happen in high school with the fair-skinned girls. She walked around with a slew of female minions that were also on the track team that just wanted to be around her because she was so beautiful. They ranged from all nationalities too. This was abnormal, since we were in Des Moines, Iowa. Although she was beautiful, she was still considered a "minority" or, a politically better word, an "African American." I wouldn't say the entire city was racist. Actually, you would see a lot of biracial people that lived off campus, originally from the city. However, I don't think it could have been a headquarters for the Black Panthers either.

In fact, there were quite a few rednecks, and they would spray-paint derogatory racial slurs on the campus buildings at times. Racism is definitely a seed related to the negative perception of body image. It teaches us that who you are is not good enough based *solely* on your outer appearance, so I am sure that that was damaging to my inner self without me even knowing it. I'm sure it was damaging to us all. It was definitely damaging to my second roommate. I began to recognize that she suffered from low self-esteem related to her dark-brown skin complexion. She didn't see herself as prettier than anyone who was lighter than she was. She never vocally said those exact words, but I could feel it, and, based on some of the things she said and did, I could confirm it to be evident. Especially how she bragged about this girl on her track team that apparently was the "Mary, mother of Joseph" to all of the girls on the track team. This was something that stuck with me because I couldn't understand her lack of love for herself.

Until, one day, she brought this beautiful stranger to our room in tears. Her once curly, lovely locks were semi-permanently straightened, and by a white girl no less. She let one of her white girlfriends go out and get a box relaxer and put it on her head. Poor thing. She was completely perplexed.

She cried to me and my roommate, "My hair is ruined. Will it go back to its original state?"

Honestly, I didn't know what to tell the girl, but, from my experience, once you get a relaxer your natural curl pattern is never the same unless you allow it to grow all the way out. Her hair was straightened and even curled with what appeared to be a wide-barrel curling iron. She was still pretty, despite the tears that stained her face, previously painted of makeup. I guess they were going out on the town or something. My roommate was trying to console her, but I could tell she was secretly getting a kick out of this girl's dismay. I assume it was a bit satisfying to see this perfect person be not so perfect by her own standards. See, low self-worth identifies with low self-worth. What already lived in my roommate found identity in what was coming out of this pretty girl's mouth and actions. This is a sad concept but unfortunately very true, especially among women.

Hell, I must say, though, I was quite perplexed myself. As I tried to assure this child that it wasn't the end of the world, I had to keep it real. So I had to ask her, with no filter attached, "Girl, why did you let this white girl do your beautiful, natural, African-American hair in the first place?"

The reason why I knew a white girl did her hair was because my roommate made it her business to mention that at the start of this catastrophic meeting. She brought this girl to me because I used to be an assistant to a hairstylist back home in Harvey, Illinois, over the summer before I went away to college. I guess she figured that made me the hair whisperer, but it didn't. Luckily, it's not rocket science to know that if you are a black girl, you probably shouldn't let your white track teammate friend relax your hair with a Dark and Lovely box relaxer from Walgreens. I mean, hell, the box alone says Dark and Lovely, and while that girl may have been lovely, she sure as hell wasn't dark. No shade to white women at all, though. I know some white girls that can set a black woman's hair off. However, they work in salons and have licenses along with the *rest* of the beauticians of *all* nationalities. I get the fact that we were all pretty poor in college and didn't have the resources to go to a salon, but come on, girl, this is a perm! These are *real* chemicals!

After I asked her that question, she replied in tears, "She said she knew what she was doing and that my hair would go back to its original state."

Now, just as much as this other girl didn't seem to know much about treatments for black women, I didn't know much about treatments or perms for white women. However, I did know that white women get perms to make their hair curly, while black women get relaxers to make their hair straight. So, maybe their hair goes back to straight over time. I replied, "In my experience, these chemicals need to grow out of your hair in order for it to return to its original state." Then I felt bad because she just started crying even more. She then gets the girl on the phone and yells at her. The girl then comes to my room like she was going to fix everything. Ironically, she did!

She came right in and looked this crying mess of a person in her face and said, "It's okay, my mom said it will go back, and you are still so beautiful either way. I know what I am doing, you will be fine."

I just sat quietly while my roommate looked on in disbelief. After pretty girl's friend came to the room (I use pretty girl as her name to avoid disclosing her identity) and said that to her, she then just nodded and left with her, like some sort of puppet. It was almost like this girl had cast a spell on her. Very interesting, I thought! I think my roommate lost a bit of respect for her at that point. I know I definitely did. I bet it was interesting to see that someone she thought was so perfect was actually a bit of a dingbat. Quiet as it's kept, I appeared to be super confident and on top of my game at the time, but I found a bit of comfort in knowing that she wasn't perfect either. She was the type of pretty that could make you question your own appearance, especially when the same guys that bowed at her feet didn't even care if you were alive. This revealed some of the insecurities of my own.

The ironic thing about this entire situation was that while we are all thinking this girl was the bomb.com, she was actually in the worst predicament. See, she needed the approval of others to feel validated. This is a dangerous thing. I mean, what happens when those people run out of compliments? I guess this would explain her entourage. They didn't really need her, though, like it seemed. Turns out she was the one who needed them, and that was sad. My roommate may have felt inadequate about her outer appearance, but I can tell you that what she felt she lacked in outer appearance, she exceeded in personality and pure inner beauty. My roommate was a smart girl and had quite a bit of depth. This girl was basically a pretty book cover, only to find that when you opened it up the pages were blank. Once again, I learned that you cannot judge a book by its cover.

Through the rest of my college years, I saw many other girls around me fall victim to body image, especially the African-American girls. There weren't many black people to begin with, and most of the black men were athletes or law students. You never saw the law students, because they had their own library and appeared to have no time for anything but their studies. The other half of black men were athletes, and they only had eyes for the white girls. I can't remember why, but I remember how it made me feel for certain. This concept began to impact how I viewed myself. I loved myself without a doubt, or so I thought, but the seeds were being watered much more often during this time.

Just as in college, today I continue to see women in the entertainment industry who view themselves as subpar. Social media has taken over this generation, and often we find ourselves comparing our outer appearance to false advertisements. Blue smoke and mirrors, in my opinion. It's difficult to get away from, when that is the way society has built its process of engaging people. It's to the point now that many people don't even have to go out of the house anymore to meet anyone. Put a few photos on Instagram or Facebook and gain interest. For some people, a few followers are more important than actual substantial interactions with human beings. It is sad to see, but it is our new truth. I had never really been one to compare my size to others. I've never thought of myself as less attractive as someone else. I just always felt like once God makes you, you are made, so work on what you have. Slowly but surely, that positive outlook would take a drastic change.

It was also around this time that I began to harvest my passion for music.

The Artist

"Let the Music Play" – Shannon

I started fostering my style and love for music as an art. I found that I loved the art of music—the history, the context, the content, and the meaning. For those very reasons, shortly after beginning college I changed my major from psychology, with a theater minor, to music education. My view of music was pure. I saw music as a newborn child sees their mother, completely untainted. Simply put, it was a form of love, an expression of art through lyrics, sounds, and melody. Music was the escape that allowed me to express myself. Everything I felt emotionally I began to release through music. My training was in classical music, which boasts singers of all shapes and sizes. I had been exposed to everything from gospel, jazz, pop, R&B, and the blues. But classical music gave me freedom to be different. I loved this learning style and the feeling of this art. Classical music allowed me to flex my love muscles. It truly became a muse for me. Singing was encouraging during my time in college. I was taken by its ability to create peace and identity in me at the same time. It later became more than art, but at that time the purity kept me exploring further into it.

Soon after diving into music, my life began to take another direction altogether. The music seeds planted as a child had been nourished by all of the beautiful sounds throughout my years, and a harvest was beginning. I transitioned my life into a musical world. Even though I thought that I loved my body and myself, nothing could prepare me for the entertainment industry obstacles I would face as a national recording artist. At this time, while

I was pursuing my degree in music, I was simultaneously striving to become a professional music star. I didn't make a big deal about it, because my confidence in music wasn't as strong as it was when sports was concerned. But I saw my father do it, and he is the closest person to me that was a living, breathing blood relative that I could identify with musically. Ironically, he was the one person that shot me down musically the most when I was a child, screaming at me for singing around the house. Telling me I couldn't sing and to literally "Shut up!" Ironically, he was the first one to take me into a studio to record my first record at fifteen years old. Go figure. I never really understood my dad. I still don't fully get him to this day.

However, after being in this game, I can see where he too may have developed insecurities as a man in the industry. He not only dealt with negative image issues, but also racism, up close and personal. He was on the road when the restrooms were marked "Colored," and the restaurants had the audacity to spell out "whites only" across the doors of their establishments, without any regard. He was on the road when the KKK burned crosses and threw bricks through the windows of black artists' tour buses. Raised on a farm in Holland Springs, Mississippi, the Deep South, encountering racism on a day-to-day basis, he didn't exactly have it easy. You could say he had a reason for some of his ill-mannered behaviors toward white industry heads. So maybe he gets a bit of a pass for his blunt way of expressing himself.

For a long time I thought I wanted to be a doctor. In many instances, I wanted to just play basketball because it was my first love. Actually, it still holds a place in my heart in many ways. After all, I did go on to marry two men who were basketball players when I met them. Contrarily, my voice took me in the direction of a record deal; I went from

Syleena the athlete, to Syleena the artist. Prior to this transition, I thought of music purely. As discussed, I really fell for the art of music, not the business.

What does that really mean? I still believe artistry should have nothing to do with what you look like. The focus should be on the artist's unique sound, or the feelings that are invoked in listeners, not on whether they are a size six and marketable for a magazine cover. When you think of the message that this sends to our children, it's actually quite sickening and discouraging. Essentially, we are saying to them, "To play this instrument, you have to be a size four, or no one will hear your music." I'd love to see a recording of their expression and the feeling that one would feel delivering that information. Just saying that to myself alone makes me want to cringe. There are so many wrongs wrapped in a package called a record deal. You think getting the deal means you have made it, but the truth is the journey has just begun. This rat race is real, and you are now officially one of the rats. What you knew as the beautiful, poetic melody of music is now called show business.

Getting signed to Jive Records was a shock to my mental system.

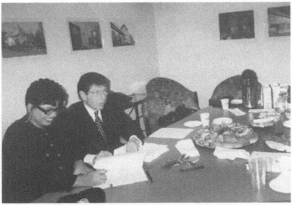

Signing contract with Alan Siegel at Jive Records, NYC 1998

My view of music started to deteriorate early on, and I didn't even know it. Every encounter with the executive team at that label for me was damaging in so many ways. I thought they were all geniuses because they held really prestigious positions and called shots when it came to the careers of megastars like R. Kelly, Britney Spears, The Backstreet Boys, Joe, NSYNC, and many others. Naturally, when they told me I needed to lose weight I thought that they were totally right, even though I was a size ten-twelve. Telling me this was a huge shock to everything I knew about myself. This very moment in my life had a spiraling effect of low self-esteem and feelings of inadequacies that sent me straight into overeating and depression. It took little to no time to figure out that this music—sound and voice—was a business. I was now faced with being the complete package, which, according to the label, included a beautiful face and a skinny waist. My voice became less and less of the focus for the label and more of an accessory to all of the other requirements. A few times I sat down and thought about whether the requirements to look wonderful were related to the genre or style of music I was in, R&B. I would look at most male artists and see there was less focus on the weight of the singer and more on the artistry. This was especially the case in the hip-hop genre. Whereas in R&B music you must be fit and beautiful to have mainstream audience appeal. Unfortunately for women in this industry, this was a silent, mandatory requirement.

For this reason alone, I began to criticize myself, constantly asking myself, "Am I the biggest girl in this industry?" The way I was trying to look on the outside did not match up with who I was on the inside. As a matter of fact, it started to impact negatively who I was. I am usually a very positive person. I often see the glass as half full. I became a new being as I tried to conform to the expectations of my label, eventually seeing the glass as half empty. All of this would be fertilizer for the seeds that had been lying dormant in my spirit since childhood. I found myself torn between two groups at the label: the A&R team that loved my voice, and the marketing team that struggled with the idea of selling my image. I wanted to impress them all, and I strived daily to do just that. I wanted to be a successful artist, and I didn't want me to be the reason why I didn't achieve that goal. Yet and still I focused on the artist more than the image. My first producer as a national recording artist on Jive Records was Bob Power. He was an amazing musician and turned out to be an awesome friend and overall man.

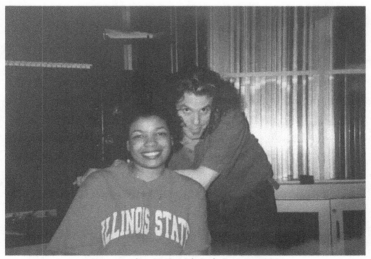

Sony studio, NYC with Bob Power 1999

I had been going through one of the worst, if not *the* worst, relationships in my personal life, and so I decided to let it bleed out through my music. I would sing these songs to Bob that I wrote, either at home, randomly out somewhere, or from my journal that I used to keep. He would then bring them to life musically. We pretty much just locked ourselves in a small writing room day after day to just vibe out. Jive would fly me into NYC to stay months at a time. Together we created the body of work that began the chapters of my life. This body of work was called *Chapter 1: Love, Pain & Forgiveness*. Creating this beautiful collage of music with him was probably one of the most pure experiences of my entire music career. He was a famous mixer and producer, while I was just a very young and naive new fish out of water, with a voice comparable to, some would say, some of the greatest female artists of our time.

Like my body, my voice developed at a very young age. I sounded the same way at sixteen and seventeen as I do now. As a matter of fact, there is a record on *Chapter 1* called "Baby I'm so Confused" that I wrote and recorded at seventeen years old. It was actually the song that was played for the CEO of the label that urged him to sign me. I later resang it for the actual LP for continuity, but it still embodied the exact same tone and emotion. I have pretty good ears and can oftentimes duplicate things pretty dead-on. I was just an artist, and he was too, even though he had been in the business for many years and was way more advanced than me in all areas. He was always respectful and viewed me as an amazing artist. He even treated me as an equal.

He was tough on me too. He wouldn't let me slack in that booth. I remember times when he had me singing until my throat was raw. At the time, I couldn't understand why, since I had pretty much produced my own vocals up until this point. However, now that I look back on it, I am glad he worked me like that. It made me a stronger and more efficient recording artist overall. My dad used to give me free rein in the studio, so I wasn't used to a whole lot of direction. But I respected Bob and looked up to him, and if I wanted to be a great leader one day, I would need to learn how to follow.

After I signed a record deal to Jive Records, my father and I had a falling out, and so I guess this was God's way of giving me a viable substitute. As a new artist on a major record label, I had a producer that was also a writer, a musician, an engineer, and a well-known mixer, all rolled up in one person. Ironically, he played one hell of a guitar too, which was the very instrument I used to sit and watch my dad play scales on as a little girl. This was a huge blessing that I wasn't even aware of at the time. Later I would have a different person for each job mentioned, which could be pretty costly. I wish I had a Bob Power in my life right now as an independent artist. He was the epitome of a true artist. I haven't spoken to him in years, but I miss him like those years were yesterday.

Through it all, he never once judged me or even mentioned a word about my outer appearance. It was all about the artistry, and I was lost in the realm of it until that album was done and ready to share with the rest of the label. Up until this point, my body was praised by everyone I knew. Therefore, I couldn't see why anyone would struggle with selling my image. However, some of the executives higher up in the marketing department made it clear they didn't think there was hope to sell my image to the markets my music would reach. As a result, I sat on the label for three years before my first album was released. All of the negative seeds that had been planted throughout childhood, high school, and college were blooming, all at the same time! First my career and now my whole life had suddenly become heavily about body image. Who would have thought the reality would be that the way that I looked would drive my career? What I was once praised for I was now rejected for. At least that is how things were perceived during this time in my life.

I took everything the label said seriously, because it was my livelihood at stake and, more than anything else, my artistry, which I had put so much work into. I desperately wanted my artistry to be shared with the world, and at its purest form. Should I conform or adapt? There are several ways you could view how I handled the situation. The obvious part is that I too gave into body image. I too needed to make the changes they requested to get the things I wanted. I did not want to sit on any label because of my weight. Subsequently, I hired a personal trainer. Unfortunately, I went completely backward in my efforts. Turns out those seeds were blooming, and depression had already started to set in.

I was living with a man who would soon become my husband, and then shortly after become my ex-husband. We were very young, and he too was dealing with some of his own demons. We had a very stressful and, at some moments, very turbulent relationship. I was frustrated from sitting on the label, and he was dealing with the passing of his mother. My first husband adored his mother. She was his best friend, and she passed away when he was nineteen. He carried the pain of her loss heavily, and when I came along I somewhat filled that void. The only problem was, I couldn't fill the void because I *never* could. A girlfriend, side chick, best friend, or even a wife can never fill the shoes of a mother.

This was one of the main reasons we consistently bumped heads. He was a really good guy. We just met up at the wrong time in life. Besides, I was no walk in the park either. I was signed in 1998 and it was the year 2000. I had been through so many ups and downs. I had even suffered from vocal cord drama that I would later make even worse.

I was sitting on this label so long, doing nothing. I had been there so long chilling that I had learned the names of every single person down to the mail room man at the label. Hell, the head of artist development and my production manager were bridesmaids in my wedding. It was a tough time in my life. Instead of transforming into this fit body of work that could sing for the gods, I transformed into an overweight ball of depression, stressed by a marriage that wasn't working and an album that was sitting. I went in complete reverse. I lost myself, as well as the fire lit by the artist inside of me, and I wasn't sure how to get her back. On my wedding day, I stood at 218 pounds and just couldn't get it together from there.

You see, when you're extremely unhappy, your sadness acts as a film that hides the reality of who you truly are as well as what is really happening. Hope is lost, and everything that is negative about you or around you becomes your new reality. You gravitate toward it even. It takes something special or traumatic to spark a light-bulb moment. So, I hired a personal trainer again and began to try and focus through the film of negativity and circumstances that now overshadowed my heart and mind. I began to transform my body into the celebrity that they originally hoped for me to be. Not only did I diet and exercise, but I took things to another level. I trained all the time, sometimes twice a day even. I would do two and three aerobics classes at the gym in one day. My poor body was sore all the time, but I was familiar with soreness because of my previous athletic days. Clearly, I was no stranger to physical pain, especially since it had the convenient ability to drown out my mental anguish.

It probably was a lot on me to handle, but I am very competitive and driven, so I just did what I thought was necessary. At this point, I figured being skinny would calculate to being happy and successful. I figured I would have more energy to be more physically romantic with my husband as well as be all that my label wanted and more. As for me, I am not sure that what I truly wanted mattered anymore. I just switched the focus to doing what was needed to achieve the obvious goal I signed up for in the first place. I had no interest in being Syleena Johnson, the artist, I now wanted to become Syleena Johnson, the famous celebrity recording star!

The Celebrity

"Overnight Celebrity" – Twista

From airbrushed photos to fad diets, everything began to surround the idea of body image. It was the real deal Holyfield of "blue smoke and mirrors," and I was right in the middle of it, trying to find my place. It's an understatement to say that I have tried it all when it comes to dieting. To keep up the image of a celebrity and be what the industry determined as suitable, I abused my body with any and everything, ranging from starvation, to diet pills, to even non-FDA-approved substances. You could safely say I could never be a professional athlete due to the substances that I had consumed. Had they tested my blood, they would have cut me before I ran my first mile on the first day of practice. I became a maniac. I had lost twenty pounds, but I was still, like, 195 pounds. I felt better and looked better, but it just never seemed like enough for others.

I then went on the TP2 tour with R. Kelly. This is where my first marriage took its most brutal beating. I was singing my brains out every night, working hard to establish myself, working an album, and trying to make everyone happy, just to come back to the bus or hotel to fight and argue with my husband. He became my tour manager at that time because the previous guy wasn't pulling his weight. My husband was very efficient at his job, but he wore me out. I understand now that he was just trying to be romantic and spend some time with his wife after the show, but I was either too tired physically or just plain ole mentally drained. Performing takes a lot out of you, so whoever you decide to be with in the industry must know this coming in the door. My first husband didn't know this was going to be the case, and neither did I. I had been in the business longer, but I had never been this busy. It was hard on him, and I suppose he was just acting out from the rejection of it all. It really angered him.

When I think about it, I realize that maybe it could have mirrored the rejection he felt when God took his mother. Now the music business was taking his wife. Eventually, this led to a separation. I did have some good memories with him. We weren't always unhappy, and I can say he never made me feel bad about being overweight. This was probably what made me want to marry him. In a time when I felt so ugly because of what I was going through, he showed an unconditional love for me, and I received it with open arms. He also encouraged fitness. That is one of the perks of dating or marrying an athlete. They take care of themselves, so they encourage you to do the same, and that is a good thing.

Shortly after we came home from the tour, I moved in with my mom, and we started the divorce proceedings. It took three years to be final, but it was inevitable. He resisted the entire three years, causing so much anguish. I used to penalize him in my heart for many years after we divorced, but then I matured and realized we were just both dangerously in love with the wrong person at the wrong time. We made silly mistakes because we were young. I'm sure he looks back on it all and feels the same way. Maturity has a sneaky way of convicting you. Previously, I talked about seeds being planted, but not all of them were negative. Good or bad, growth is the ultimate goal, and despite it all, I was growing up.

Meanwhile, my first nationally released album, *Chapter 1: Love, Pain and Forgiveness*, had been worked to its capacity and it was time to move on to the next chapter, which later became *Chapter 2: The Voice*. I had bounced back quite a bit after my divorce, with the help of prayer and fasting. Some fragments of that negative film that hovered over me had been lifted and I was on the road to loving myself again. I had gotten down in weight a bit more and started working my second album. I would go on to have my biggest hit from that album, called "Guess What," and suddenly I was a credible artist with a promising future. After the success of *Chapter 2*, I would then begin to record *Chapter 3: The Flesh*.

I suddenly had this bright idea. I experienced some great success from *Chapter 2*, but I wasn't exactly where I wanted to be physically. I figured it was because I *still* wasn't pretty enough or skinny enough, from my distorted view. So, I decided that I was going to find a way to make everyone see that this body type was marketable.

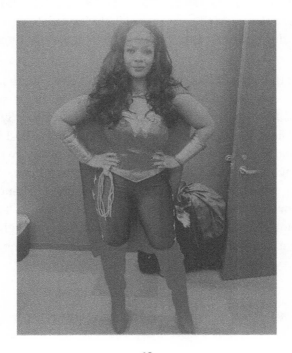

I began to do research, and I came across a book I found in Barnes & Noble that had Wonder Woman on the front. I opened it up to see that it was a book praising her body as well as several other Amazon women. It talked about the women in Greek mythology and how they were great and powerful warriors. It explained how they were not only warriors, but they were very beautiful and intelligent, with bodies that were praised like works of art. This was my proof! I was determined to find the positive in being five ten, 180 pounds. Their bodies were muscular and toned, and the average weight of them ranged from 145 pounds to 170 pounds. These women were beautiful, strong, and confident. They were everything I used to be. However, at this time in my life, I felt I was not. So, I had the bright idea of dropping an additional twenty to twenty-five pounds so that I could emulate this idea of being an Amazon and proud of it. I even referred to it as being a "Glamazon." I used the theme of this concept to help formulate my album cover design for *Chapter 3*, which I later boldly titled *The Flesh.*

At this point, I had every intention of showing that flesh too. I was fed up with feeling inadequate about what I looked like. I was going to make them notice me, Syleena, the athlete, because this was the girl that not only I loved, but that everyone else seemed to think was pretty awesome too. I even inked a modeling deal with Wilhelmina modeling agency, which was one of the largest modeling agencies in the world. It was the full-figured division, of course. I mean, let's not get ahead of ourselves. I may have thought that being a glamazon was the new skinny, but the modeling industry *definitely* did not.

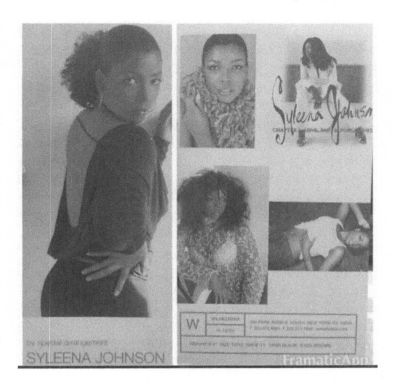

The modeling world is an entirely different beast. You literally had to look like you hadn't eaten in several years to be a straight-size model. And as for your feelings, they were unbothered and unfiltered. They would flat out tell you eyeballs to eyeballs that you were too fat, too short, not the right look, boring, bland, and basically never going to make it in life. You had to have alligator skin to be a straight-size model, which was size zero to size four, with four being on the heavy side. I believe this was the case because most of the sample sizes were twos and zeros. They would say that was the reason, but I suspect there was more to it than that.

It wasn't like that in the full-figured division. They praised you for being a size ten and up. At the time I was a size six-eight, but I was still considered to be full-figured. I didn't care. I wanted to be a model, and model meant beautiful in my eyes and most of the eyes in the world. Plus, they thought I was beautiful, because they told me so. They wouldn't have signed me if that wasn't the case, right? In addition, this deal could help me gain some press from another outlet, because my label seemed to be struggling in that area. Now, am I the pretty girl from college who needed outside validation? Wow. It's funny how the tables turn. Eventually, outside validation would be my personal formula for achieving self-love. This was when my seeds bloomed into full-grown flowers, honey, but, unfortunately, with a sizable number of weeds. I was lost.

The reality of the music business is that we put ourselves out there *just* for you to judge us. In most cases, our entire existence is built on whether or not you the consumer think we are good enough. This is a great job, and I am grateful to God that he has given me this gift to share with others, but sometimes I wish I had a different job. In reality, that could never be the case for me, though. I love music so much. I am not sure how I would survive without it.

This is when the diet pills and the dangerous starving started again. I would fast for nine and ten days straight. Basically, I was borderline anemic. I took any and every diet pill known to mankind. I trained three times a day. Sometimes I would sleep in the gym and just go home after the last workout, which was a nighttime Tae Bo class. I would leave my house at 6 a.m., and not return until 10 p.m., because the last workout class was at 8 p.m. My trainer was a drill sergeant. He was, and still is, a fitness competitor, so he knew how to get me to where I needed to be, and that is just what he did. He singlehandedly shaped my body into probably the best body I had had in my life. I got down to 165 pounds of muscle and very low body fat. I felt like Serena Williams or Laila Ali or somebody. I felt strong, and most of the time I thought I was beautiful—most of the time.

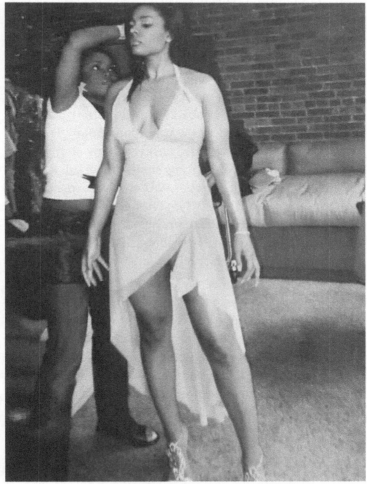

Chapter 3 album jacket photo shoot 2004

Ironically, I would still look in the mirror and think I was too big. So, I continued to starve to make sure I didn't gain any weight. This is clearly a disorder called "body dysmorphia." I not only recognized it in myself, but I saw it in my sisters and close girlfriends as well. You see, even though they weren't in the entertainment industry, they were still subject to the criticism if they were seen or associated with me. This was very unfair. It basically says that not only do you have to be flawless, but you must only be seen with flawless people. Talk about pressure? Talk about carrying a heavy weight? This was the height of it.

Eventually, they too would become weight conscious and diet maniacs as well, and I guess part of that is my fault. I developed migraines, probably from the horrible eating and the terrible substances I was putting into my body, not to mention the amount of stress I was putting on myself. In addition, I was on a very strong birth control pill that was designed to manage my acne. I was on a roll, so I couldn't have my face go crazy while I had lost all of this weight. My face stayed clear, even though my blood vessels were taking a beating. I didn't know much about that, nor did I care. I just wanted to be beautiful and successful.

I was single and loved the attention. I was a *celebrity*. I dated athletes and walked red carpets. I even became a bit of a party girl. I thought it was feeding my self-esteem in a positive way, when all it really did was reward my negative ways of getting to the goal. Going through this misery was what it took to get there, but what was it going to take to stay there? I developed acid reflux and it took a toll on my voice. I struggled daily just to talk in the mornings. I saw countless ENT (ear, nose, and throat) doctors until one put me on Nexium. I didn't want to take any more pills, but what the hell, I had already taken many others by now, so whatever. I couldn't have my voice go out on me when I finally got to "the goal." Clearly, everything around me was suffering, but at least I was cute, according to Jive. Well, to some of them.

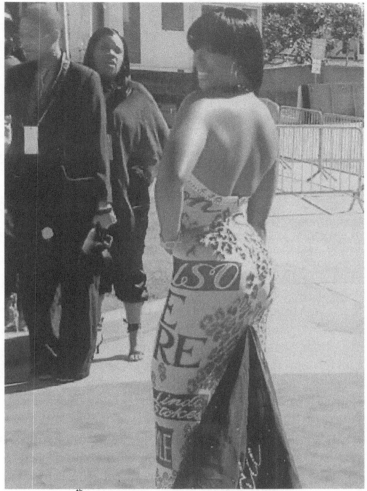

9th Annual Soul Train Lady of Soul Awards 2003

The label seemed to be happy with my new look, and some of them even made positive comments about it. During this time, I was able to collaborate with Kanye West on what would later become his debut hit record. This was an awesome time in my life. He took me everywhere with him to help promote that record, and it helped create lots of awareness for me. It woke the label up as well.

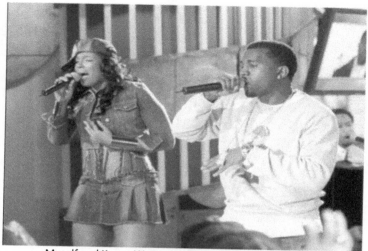

Myself and Kanye West on MTV Total Request Live 2004

They had always been kind of mild when it came to me, but this gave them a reason to really work *Chapter 3: The Flesh*, so I thought. After working the Kanye record, I was ready for *Chapter 3* to drop! I just knew I had done everything I could have possibly done. Many people tried to convince me that my fans were not going to believe in my music if I didn't look the part. This mentality changed my approach to music as a career. This mentality changed how I viewed music altogether: it was no longer this pure artistry; it was my livelihood at stake. Conforming to meet standards of the labels and others was something I had to do to see the success I wanted in my career. This is how my mind was conditioned over and over again. This is how I was able to jeopardize everything, including my voice, just to weigh in at 165, just to prove that I was beautiful at this height and weight. I was trying very hard to match an image of Greek mythology and thinking that was going to create an ah-ha moment for the record executives. This was foolish thinking at its finest. Truthfully, most record executives don't care what you look like or sound like. The question is, can you make money?

I became extremely moody, and there were a few things that could be said that would trigger my attitude immediately. This is far from my true personality. I used to be very shy and reserved. I know that is pretty hard to believe about me now, but that was indeed the case. The effects of the industry sent my personality and level of patience down the drain.

The sad thing is, I probably could have resolved many of my personality issues with a donut, but I had an image to keep up, and carbs were a no-no. My fasting and starvation stints went from days to weeks at a time. I would go to a club on promotional opportunities and drink liquor on an empty stomach, continuing the trend of unhealthy dieting habits. The lifestyle of a celebrity often entails late nights at the club, but my stamina to keep up this type of schedule and look good meant a mix of energy drinks, diet pills, early morning exercise, and small-portion eating—a clear-cut recipe for disaster. Some people have a hard time sticking to one thing; I was doing everything all at once.

When my mind is set on things, I go extra hard to get the results I am looking for. My mentality was to treat "celebrity" as a match or a tournament. Each photo and video became game day, and I was working out and training to prepare for the next photo shoot or video. The behavior I was demonstrating was very similar to an athlete on game day. I went all week long working toward a physical goal. I would fast and dehydrate myself to ensure I looked perfect. Perfect being the key word here—a word that no one on earth can achieve. Nonetheless, I was striving for perfection, and no one in my life could steer me away from that bumpy and unrealistic path. Everything, including the weight loss, came at a cost.

What I viewed as "blue smoke and mirrors" had now become a way of life. I was in a whirlwind of fad diets and celebrity expectations. I didn't care about my overall health. I never stopped to celebrate my body and how I looked throughout the progression of my career. I was too busy maintaining the upkeep of being a celebrity. That lack of celebration created a routine of getting used to mental hardship while adapting to these unhealthy routines. If I wasn't suffering in some form or fashion, I wasn't winning.

Meanwhile, the album that I thought would take me to the mountaintop would unfortunately cause further depression and stress. *Chapter 3* was finished, the Kanye West single "All Falls Down" was at the top of the charts, and my hopes were extremely high. I did everything, from research, to starving, to damn near dying, so the rest was on the record label. Since I viewed them as geniuses, I knew I could not lose. After all, they had made at least 80 percent of their artists' megastars, so what could possibly be the problem? Even though I felt like this, I wasn't happy. I wanted everyone else around me to believe that this was going to be *the* moment that my career went to the next level, but did I truly believe it? After all the blood, sweat, and tears I had shed to get to this point, I thought I would feel differently. Strangely, I felt a huge void and didn't understand why. I guess I was the perfect person to be on Kanye's song.

Things clearly started to all fall down for me after the release of *Chapter 3*. Needless to say, it didn't do as well as I'd hoped. It actually did worse than the previous album, and I wasn't a size six like I was for this album. Now that I look back on it all, I can tell you exactly why. The problem was that I sold my happiness for success, only to find that they are not equal in value. Actually, they are not even in the same category. Happiness must be the reason *why* you are successful, and not the other way around. When you are truly happy inside, you are satisfied with you on all levels, and you are at peace within. The light from within shines bright through your spirit, and others are attracted to it naturally. Choosing to be happy and who God made you to be brings his favor and blessings. This is when true success can have an opportunity to plant itself in your life. There is so much more to life, and I hadn't even begun to achieve any of it. I would come home from being on the road and sadly notice that I was alone. I could call out my own name in my two-bedroom townhome and hear no one answer but an echo. I was alone. No man, no kids, no foundation, and no one to share the fruits of my labor with. The void that I felt would soon be filled on May 26, 2005, when I met the love of my life, Kiwane Garris.

The Wife

"He Loves Me" – Jill Scott

I was still working and maintaining my figure, but I was starting to notice more and more that I was alone and, subsequently, very lonely. After recording *Chapter 3*, I met my husband, Kiwane Garris. Meeting him would change my perception of love forever. However, before we jump into all of the great things Kiwane has brought to my life, I have to say the journey of getting to him was quite difficult.

When I look back on the choices I made on men in the past, I can connect those choices to how I felt about myself during that time. It is true we are what we attract. Prior to meeting Kiwane, I wasn't solid inside, so I picked broken men. They, in turn, ended up breaking my heart and worsening what was already a growing problem. I remember dating a guy who was also famous in his own right, and when it came to him and me, we kept our relationship pretty private. Sometimes it seemed like the relationship was nonexistent, like it wasn't real. I never knew why, really. I assume it was probably because we were so on-again, off-again.

There was one incident I will never forget. I asked him to walk with me on the red carpet at the BET awards. I had no date, and I wanted people to know that we were together. I was ready to go public with our relationship. I guess I was thinking that would make it real. Apparently, we weren't on the same page, because he easily declined. I remember wondering if the decline was because he had other women and didn't want them to see, or because he didn't think I was a big enough star to walk with, in comparison to him. Now that may have been my own insecurities, but he was very Hollywood like that, so it wouldn't have been farfetched. Maybe that is why we never quite made it. I am a very down-to-earth girl on the inside. I loved the limelight at that time and would definitely turn it on when it was time, but with my man I was the housewife type. Up until this day I still am. That rejection jumped to many other conclusions as well, and you could just about guess how it made me feel. Granted, during that time he was a popular athlete and our relationship was on the low, but never once did I think he would decline an invitation to something that would show support for me and my career, especially since I had flown in for his games on many occasions.

For three years, I put myself through an on-again, off-again, meaningless fiasco, and no one knew of it. I adored him, though. He was a Southern boy from South Carolina, and when we were together he was always a gentleman and very respectful. He seemed mysterious but intriguing to me at that time. I was fascinated by him and loved how strong he was as a man. He told me he wasn't the limelight type. I believed in him and whatever he said.

Now that I look back on it, I realize—he was just full of shit. I knew it all along. He wasn't ready for a serious relationship, and I was. I heard from others later on that he may have even had several women he was dating in addition to me at that time, which was *not* the understanding. Or, maybe he was just stringing me along simply because I let him. Men do that in relationships all the time. Hell, I know women who do it; it's not unheard of. I will never know, and luckily it will never matter. Either way, it doesn't make him a bad person or me a victim. It just made us both selfish at that time. Him for not keeping it 100 percent with me about his true feelings, and me for not letting go of something because of the short satisfaction it intermittently gave.

Needless to say, no parts of this concept equaled to a healthy relationship with him, or with myself, for that matter. In hindsight, one could say it was a complete waste of time, but I can't thank him enough for showing me what *not* to accept in a love relationship. The pain he caused me inspired some really great records. So, actually, it wasn't a total waste. Having a bad experience prepares you for the good ones. I could run down a list of things that I found in men that I didn't care for in a relationship, but this book is about learning to love *me* and not others. Besides, I can't love others until I love me anyway.

I learned that the perception I created of myself was driving my negative attraction to others. I was attracting beautiful specimens carrying heavy, dirty loads of baggage. This was an exact mirror image of who I was at the time, and I didn't even know it. Yes, I had gotten my body and outer appearance right where I wanted it, but my insides were all a mess. Ironically, I wondered why none of these relationships worked out. Clearly, I was perpetuating my own issues by allowing people to dig into existing wounds. As long as doubt existed within me about myself, I would allow for others to dismiss my wants and needs. This cycle needed to end, and I needed to be the person to end it.

Who would have known that the ending would start with a phone call from a close friend? I had just returned from a long trip filled with back-to-back performances, and I was so tired. Not only was I physically tired, I was also mentally tired and frankly over the whole dating scene. This call would be different. This call would change my entire world as I knew it. It would fill my cup until it overflowed, all the way up to this very day.

I got a call from my friend Dave, whose girlfriend worked with the twin cousins of a guy who played basketball overseas, and this basketball player apparently wanted to take me out on a date. That guy was Kiwane Garris.

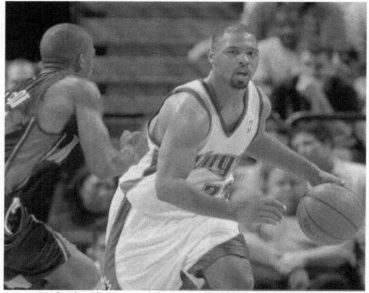

My husband Kiwane while playing for the Sacramento Kings

The first thing I thought was, *Oh God, here we go again, another athlete.* Lately, that had been all that I had attracted, and, honestly, I was over them. Around this time, I had taken a vacation from dating, and I really wasn't in the mood for more heartbreak. I was trying to focus on the release of *Chapter 3*, and I didn't think I could do that with a man in my life, especially if he was going to act a fool.

My friend Dave insisted that this guy was a good guy and that I should reach out to him. So, I Googled him. I needed to know if he was an ax murderer, his age, his height (which is very important to me since I am so tall), what he looked like, and whatever else I could find out about him. I am a huge sports fan and I had heard of him from my college years, but I wasn't real familiar with him. To my pleasant surprise, he was very handsome and older than me. He was also born in the same month as me, but he was a Libra. I am very into astrological signs, so finding out when he was born was key. Libras are cool, and I tend to do well with them, so his resume was checking out.

Finally, after a full recon of who he was, I decided to tell Dave to just go ahead and give him my number. He called me that same day, and we set a date to go to dinner for two days later. That day was Thursday, May 26, 2005, to be exact. He was so handsome when I met him. He was tall and clean-cut, but he was a little shy and laid back. He had on a linen suit and Air Force Ones for our first date. I remember it like yesterday, because I was totally unbothered. I showed up in a BEBE jogging suit that had DANGEROUS printed across my bottom. He probably should have run for the hills then, but he didn't. He just smiled, looking damn near albino with his fair-colored skin and light-brown goatee.

No matter how fine he was to me, I didn't allow myself to show any emotion. I gave him a friendly hello, a chest-only touch hug, and proceeded to get in the passenger seat of his Denali. I had a blonde-and-brown weave in my head, hazel-green contacts (they were in style at the time), and Louis Vuitton flip-flops. I was *definitely* sending the message that I was an around the way girl from Harvey, Illinois, and did not care one bit. I know he was probably expecting "Syleena Johnson," but I was getting a bit tired of her. So, I tried my luck with just Syleena, or Leena, which is what my close family and friends know me by.

Normally when I went out on a date with a guy, I would dress up in heels and makeup and try and look the part. I would turn the "Syleena Johnson" volume all the way up. I would try and exude confidence through who she was and what she had accomplished. I would use my celebrity as my own personal boost of confidence.

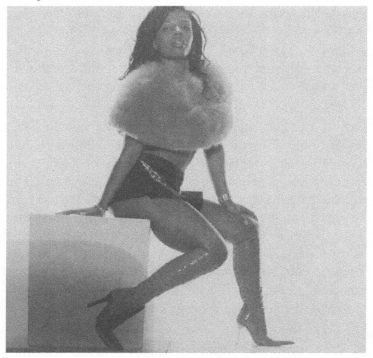

Body image was intact, but I struggled tremendously trying to hide this monster inside of me. I didn't have the strength to deal with all of that at this time. This time I was going to be as close to my true self as possible. At least, what I knew to be my true self.

We went to the Cheesecake Factory. He was pretty quiet the whole way, with casual conversation initiated by me sparingly throughout the evening. I have always been pretty nosy, so why stop now? Plus, it was our first date. I needed to know the goods! We sat down and ordered our food. He had the chicken piccata, and I don't remember what I had, probably because it was nasty, and I ate out of his plate *and* drank his drink the entire time. Very annoying, I must say, but it didn't bother him. Actually, he thought it was funny and encouraged me to keep eating, and I sure did. I must admit, I came across extremely ghetto and aggressive with my own views and wants, but I think subconsciously I was trying to push him away. I was tired of being hurt and confused, and I just didn't think he would appreciate me past this date anyway. The results with other guys in the past told that story, and I wasn't sure I was ready to open up a new book.

We went back and forth a bit more in casual conversation, then he paid for the meal and we left. On the way home, I fell asleep on him, mouth open and all. Now, after that, I don't know if I would have kept fooling with me, but the following Wednesday he called me and asked me to go to lunch. Lunch? Lunch was a good look. I had been used to a very trifling lifestyle when it came to men. Don't get me wrong, I wasn't promiscuous at all, but I didn't get "lunch" calls. I got either dinner or past 11 p.m. calls.

You see, that's what happens when your best foot forward isn't your mind and personality. My best foot forward was my outer appearance. I felt that since that is what everybody else in the music industry cared about, then men that pursued me were no exception to the rule. I would wear provocative clothing, and everything about my body language spoke sexual persuasions, because *lunch* was never on the menu.

Luckily, this time it was. I liked that he asked. It was a small thing, but I liked it, which led me to start liking him. I declined, though. I told him I had to work out. Still testing him, still going against the grain. I wanted someone to want me regardless of my schedule. I wanted someone who would make concessions for me. I believed that chivalry was still alive, and I was going to find it or be single forever.

I did, however, tell him I could meet him later. I invited him to my Wednesday night Bible study class. He said no at first, but I wasn't that bothered; I figured as much. Then he called me right back and decided to go. Now *that* was damn near foreplay.

After that date, we continued to go on several more. No sex, no kissing even, and he would always bring me home at a decent hour. He showed so much respect, and I was really starting to learn that someone can like you for who you are. I didn't feel like "Syleena Johnson" when I was with him. I felt like a woman who was adored by a man who was genuine and chivalrous. It was such a breath of fresh air. He was funny, handsome, sweet, and showed love for me. That's all I really wanted, and all I really needed.

That entire summer of 2005 we were inseparable. We eventually fell head over heels in love. He played basketball in Bologna, Italy, at the time, and I would happily fly four thousand miles across the water to be with him, despite my career being in full effect. At the time, my career was a symbol of stress and pressure. It always felt like I was walking around with heavy weights attached to my body or carried in my purse. Kiwane was the total opposite. He represented the freedom of that weight, and I was in a happy place. I had forgotten all about being sad and taking diet pills to get skinny. As a matter of fact, I stopped taking diet pills altogether. He didn't put that kind of pressure on me to look a certain way. He would constantly tell me how beautiful I was from what he saw on the outside as well as on the inside. He also used to say things like, "I don't like really thin women." This was very new to me. I mean, how could this be? A male athlete who wasn't interested in the thin model stereotypical armpiece chick? Wow! This opened up a whole new perspective to me.

It said to me, loud and clear: "HELLO, YOU DON'T HAVE TO BE A SIZE TWO TO BE LOVED AND ACCEPTED BY SOMEONE!"

It suddenly dawned on me that everything I had been thinking about love and how it is achieved was wrong. I wasn't loving myself, therefore no one I dated before Kiwane knew how to love me either. I have learned that you have to teach people how to treat you, and I hadn't been doing that at all. Maybe wearing that jogging suit, holding out on sex, and eating out of his plate showed him more than I thought. Maybe it said to him, "Hey, this is me, so if you want to be with me, here is the real deal," and apparently that was just what he wanted.

Being loved this way was a weird feeling at first, but I eventually got used to it. However, after September 13, 2005, *Chapter 3: The Flesh* was released, and it was hard being in a relationship of love and fighting the sadness that that release brought to my heart. I had been praying and believing that this album would do great things. I had lost tons of weight and posed damn near naked throughout the entire album jacket. I had features from some of the greatest artists in the industry then and still today. This album was supposed to catapult my career to new heights! It sold *fewer* copies than my last album, and I was devastated. I couldn't even hide my emotions from Kiwane. I just kept wondering, *How could this be?* I did everything I was supposed to do and more. It was painful.

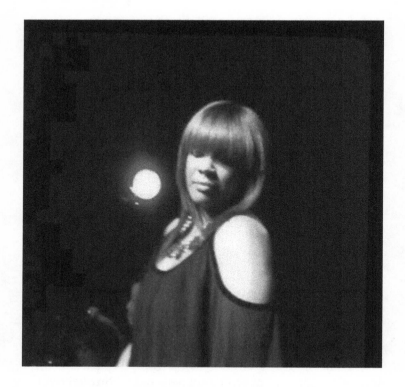

This is the point in my life where those seeds became full-blown trees. I fell into a deep depression. I cried. I stayed in bed. Then I cried some more. All of those negative emotions, all of those negative feelings came rushing back to the surface, and I had to deal with them head-on. Then the tornado hit my heart and ego at the same time.

Shortly after I tried very hard to work *Chapter 3*, Jive Records decided not to pick up the option to resign me to the label. Although I understood that this working relationship wasn't working, it still broke my heart into pieces. They were all that I had known, as far as my career was concerned, since 1998, and here we were in 2006. Eight years of trying to impress them. Eight years of fighting for an imaginary goal. But worse than anything, an eight-year decline in my self-esteem and self-worth, which caused a dramatic incline in my self-hate. They didn't even have the decency to tell me that was their decision. They just stopped the Syleena Johnson business and sent everything Syleena-like to my sister's house. They didn't even have my address or have the guts to call and ask. I had no label, no job really, a declining record, and all of these issues left to deal with. I was so sad. Just sitting here telling you about this waters my eyes.

However, there was one huge difference from when the negative seeds of the past were planted. The very moment when my world was in dismay, God sent me an angel to help me through the storm. That angel was Kiwane, who was there for me in ways that pages in a book can't fully describe. He endured my bad dreams that caused sleepless nights and tear-stained pillows that he willingly laid his head on right next to me every night. He held me through anxiety attacks and he encouraged me whenever I spoke negatively about myself. In fact, he continued to shower me with love and positive reinforcements. Subsequently, I gained twenty pounds.

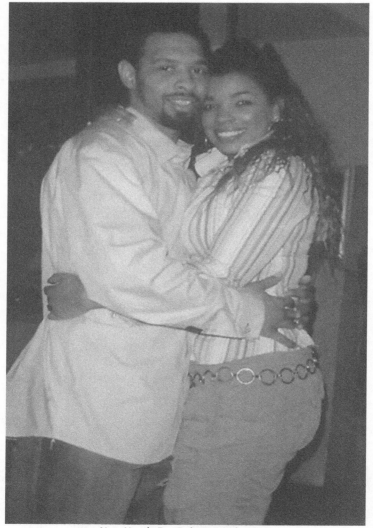

New Year's Eve Bologna, Italy 2005

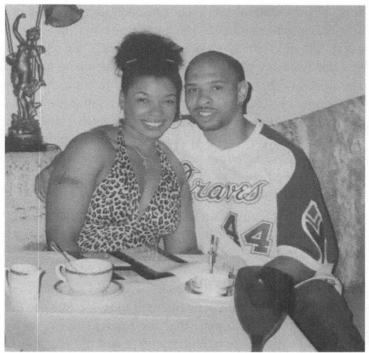

Las Vegas, 2006

I was 204 pounds when I hit bottom and cried to him for help. He called his agent, and his agent gave him the name Julie Burns, who was the dietitian for the Chicago Bulls, Bears, Black Hawks, White Sox, and Northwestern University athletes. My primary problem wasn't that I didn't know how or want to work out. My primary problem was that I didn't know how to *eat*. I had been starving and taking supplements to cheat my way to losing weight in short periods of time. This is how yo-yo dieting starts. Instead, I should have been eating clean and creating a lifestyle that would ensure optimal health for the rest of my life.

Meeting Julie was one of the best things that ever happened to me. She taught me about organic food and the benefits of healthy, natural supplementation as well as all sorts of information that I had not been privy to. She not only taught me what to eat, she taught me when and how to eat it. She did nutrition planning specifically for my body. She ran urine and blood tests and even a test on my thyroid. She was very thorough, and I was elated to learn all of the things about my body she discovered through these tests. I learned that I have dairy sensitivities, which caused my acne breakouts, and I learned that I was low in vitamin D as well as magnesium, which perpetuated the headaches I was having, as well as chronic fatigue. She taught me about iodine and its many beneficial health properties.

On the first eating plan she put me on, I lost twenty-two pounds in six weeks, eating my brains out. I ate every two and a half to three hours, and it wasn't just broccoli pops. She encouraged me to eat fat! Yep, that's right, fatty foods. However, they were good fats, like salmon, avocados, organic hotdogs, and an assortment of nuts, etc. She doesn't even truly know the impact that she has had on my entire life and now my entire family. My voice and my mood even got better. I was starting to change my focus to a positive, more relaxed mindset when it came to fitness.

Some months went by, and Kiwane and I grew even closer together. We are Christians, believing in the Lord wholeheartedly, and read His word together, trying our best to live by it each day. I would go to church and share with him the sermon via telephone, and we would read spiritual books together. He was my best friend and my personal portion of peace. When I was with him or talking to him, I was at peace. I couldn't believe that God had blessed me this way. I started to feel satisfied and full. I started the process of finding self-love with him. Loving him dearly was one thing I definitely did, but to watch him *love me* through my pain gave me permission to love me so much more.

He loved me with no exceptions, and on July 1, 2006, he proved how deep that love was. He got on one knee and asked me to marry him, presenting me with a six-and-a-half-carat diamond ring. Needless to say, I happily said yes.

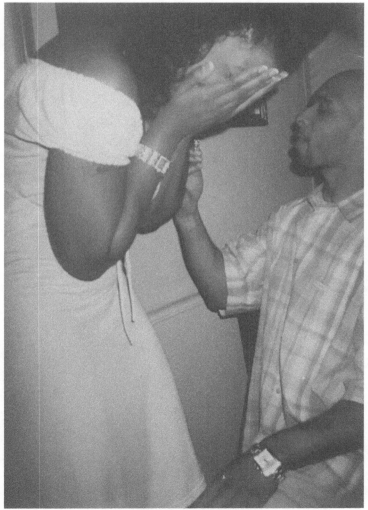

Kiwane proposed on July 1, 2006

The love inside of me had begun to heal my broken heart. We now have two beautiful children of our own, one beautiful stepson from his previous marriage, and eleven years of marriage under our belt.

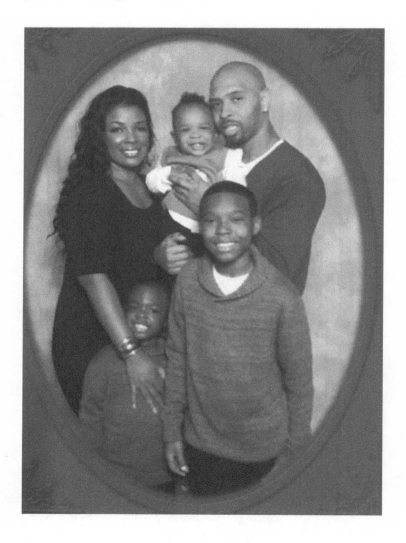

Unfortunately, through each pregnancy I gained fifty-plus pounds, but despite the weight gain, Kiwane still loved my body through every change. The love Kiwane has given me made it much easier to bounce back from each pregnancy. It also helped that I had those health tip jewels that Julie instilled in me before my pregnancy. She was also instrumental in helping me through my pregnancies.

I began the journey of loving myself, but when someone else loves you without conditions or requirements the benefit is unlimited. Many women maintain their bodies prior to having children but don't get the support they need after the child is born to bounce back. That support is instrumental from your loved ones to help you mentally stay focused. In my case, I had a real man to love all of me and support me, no matter what the circumstances. I learned through the love in my union how to love myself again. I was beginning to be okay with my imperfections, and, in his eyes, I was perfect for him.

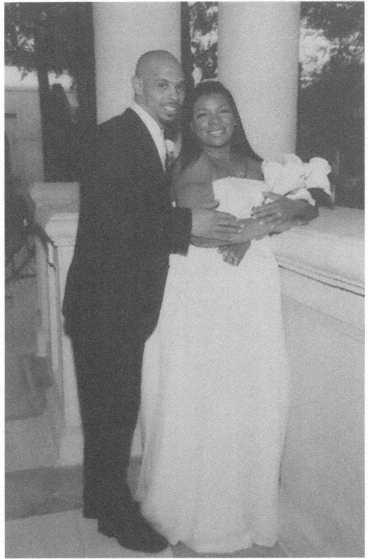

Our wedding day July 1, 2007, Bellagio Las Vegas,
eight months pregnant with KJ

One thing I have learned about real love is that it feels
the same at any size, at any weight, with any hairstyle, and

at any age. Love doesn't just flee when there are changes in physical appearance or health issues. People who love you go through the battles along with you. My husband runs with me, works out with me, diets with me, pushes through the weight loss struggle with me. Further, he supports and coaches me to be the best version of myself. He upgrades me.

When God brought this man into my life, it changed for the better forever. Now it is up to me to continue this journey of self-acceptance. From here seems like a pretty good place to start.

The Mother

"Thanks for My Child" – Cheryl Pepsii Riley

My children are my everything, and everything that I have been through has caused me to protect them from making the same mistakes that I made. As a mother, we have innate behavior that causes us to go into protection mode. We often try our hardest to keep our children from making our past mistakes. Sometimes this works, ofttimes it does not. Either way, it is our job to try. Since it took me so long to get the memo about optimal nutrition and the truth about it, I go to the extreme with my family. I am constantly educating them about nutrition and feeding them things that I didn't incorporate in my everyday eating regimen until I got to college. With food becoming increasingly more dangerous and less nutritious, it has been hard to maintain a healthy household. Luckily, I have learned so much about nutrition that my passion for it keeps me searching for information to stay up-to-date.

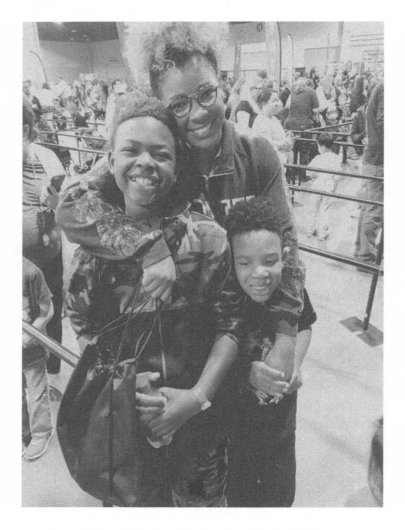

As I spoke of earlier, in my house growing up, food was associated with love. So, overeating was over-loving, and how could over-loving ever be a bad thing? Like I stated previously, we were encouraged to clean our plates. This caused negative eating habits in me, so I intend to change that with my children. As a matter of fact, after I gave birth to my first son, I began to get really serious about nutrition.

I later took that passion to a whole new level by earning my bachelor's degree in nutrition science from Kaplan University.

Body image pokes its ugly head in all areas of my life. When I was pregnant with my first child, I constantly worried about the outer aftermath of pregnancy, like stretch marks and a C-section scar. And even though saggy breasts and swollen feet plagued my dreams, I was still very determined to breastfeed.

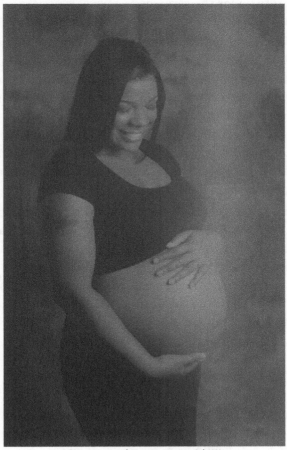

Seven months pregnant with KJ

I researched every option for my child, but breastfeeding was always the best option. In article after article, it was consistently proven that overall health and wellness for my baby now, and as he continued to grow, was connected to breastfeeding. I even read about how breastfeeding can help prevent obesity even later in their lives as adults! Clearly, I was trying to prevent obesity in my children before they even arrived. Body image surfaces over and over again, and in this context, I didn't want my children to suffer the same body image issues that I did as an adult, so breastfeeding was the move. Besides, it was free.

I was just trying to do my best as a mother so that they could live their best possible life. Meanwhile, I couldn't help but consider what my children would be exposed to, just for being mine. As a mother, you try to avoid every potential pitfall your children could endure, but the more you prepare, the more curveballs you can expect. Sometimes you just have to do the best you can and let God do the rest. Then there are other times where being a mom is really hard and you just have to do the work.

There was a time when my family was exposed to mold while we were living in Italy. This exposure created additional yeast in my son KJ's body, and of course he developed an allergy to mold. He was only two years old at the time. Prior to figuring out the real problem, I began using every home remedy I knew of at the time. The symptoms consisted of excessive ear infections, skin rashes, runny noses, and watery eyes. They were so bad that they got to the point that they were an everyday thing for my KJ. I tried every home remedy I could think of to treat my son's symptoms. Notice I said symptoms, because I wasn't really sure what was going on. There was one point in my daily research of nutrition that I discovered that various foods could prevent a child from getting sick or cure some of the symptoms naturally. Around that time, I started exposing KJ to all types of foods to ward off his symptoms as well as to prevent future illnesses. Some great things came out of that exposure, including the fact that KJ became a very diverse eater.

A year later I would find out that I was pregnant with my second child, who would later show me that being a diverse eater was not part of the plan God had for him.

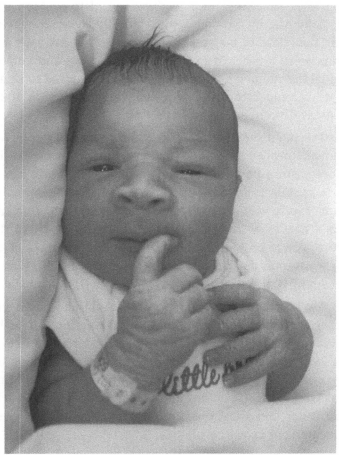

February 6, 2011 Kingston Li Garris is born

79

My second child, Kingston Li Garris, was born February 6, 2011. Everything was all good until he turned twelve months. I will never forget the day Kingston's eating behavior started to change a bit. It was shortly after he suffered from a febrile seizure after he was given his twelve-month shots. I was sitting in the stands at a basketball game that my husband was coaching, and I noticed that Kingston was very hot. Now, I had given him Tylenol at the doctor's office after his shots, like normal, but since KJ never suffered from a high fever after his shots. I didn't even think to put Motrin in his baby bag. My mother instinct quickly kicked in when I held him close to me and could feel how hot his back and arms were. I reached inside of his baby bag and got his digital thermometer, which immediately lit up red to signal that his temperature was in a high zone, reading at 102.5 degrees Fahrenheit.

I then noticed I had no Motrin and no more Tylenol, so I immediately left the game and took him with me to the grocery store down the street, so that I could give him a dose as soon as possible. I had no idea how dangerous his temperature was, but my heart knew that it wasn't safe and that I needed to move with urgency. As I pulled into the grocery store parking lot, I jumped out to get him out of his car seat—only to find him lifeless and gagging. He wasn't breathing right. Something was very wrong with my baby.

My heart stopped, and a panic started that I had never experienced before. It took over my whole body. Was he choking? What is wrong with my baby? I started to scream for help, and what had seemed like an empty parking lot became filled with just the amount of help I needed. God was with us, and in an instant the guardian angels on earth that watch and protect us, from a subliminal point of view, appeared out of nowhere.

One man came to my aid and very softly gave Kingston the Heimlich maneuver until he threw up and started crying. I had given him some crackers before we left, so I thought maybe he was choking. I wasn't exactly sure that was the case, but I was just very grateful to hear him crying.

Another lady came out of nowhere with a cell phone and called the ambulance, then another lady got on her knees and started praying with me. This all happened at once. God's presence was there, and I could feel it as clear as the Midwest cold weather that hugged my face while I drowned in fear and desperation. It was a glimpse of peace in my own personal storm. I was alone, but the feeling of his presence was assurance.

Soon the ambulance showed up, and the paramedic took his temperature, which was now at 104, and he immediately gave him Motrin. They then proceeded to hook him up to an IV and give him fluids. He was a bit lethargic, but coherent. I was in tears, frantically trying to reach Kiwane.

Moments after Kingston's fever broke, Kiwane made it there and I started to calm down. The paramedic then began to explain to us that it appeared Kingston had experienced a febrile seizure. He went on to explain that a febrile seizure is a fever-induced seizure that is common in babies until they turn five or six years old. There is no known reason why one child would be more prone to them than the other, but because the duration of them is so short, there is likely never any permanent damage. The word "seizure" put me in an uneasy place as I listened to the paramedic while watching Kingston's every breath.

Kingston then sat up and seemed to be his normal self. His fever was all the way down to 98.7, and he was smiling and moving around as usual. We did ride with him to the hospital to take further tests, but everything was normal.

The following week, we went to a neurologist to get him checked out, just in case the doctors were wrong, but he also declared that everything was normal.

Kingston would have two more febrile seizures after that day. One came six months later, and another four years later, but both while in my arms. Probably the scariest moments in my life.

The one thing that I can be thankful for, besides his overall health, is the fact that when he had those seizures he was with me the entire time. What if he had been at school? What if he were with a sitter? I would have felt worse because I wasn't there to comfort him. I would have worried myself to death trying to understand how it could have been prevented. At least this way, I know for a fact that when his fever hit, we did all we could to stop it from spiking. However, I am still trying to figure out why God had me endure that kind of emotional trauma. I'm still trying to learn the lesson.

Nonetheless, I learned quite a bit about myself in this era of motherhood. I learned just how much I can take under extreme pressure. From the first seizure on, I was constantly on guard when it came to Kingston. If it looked like he was going to sweat too much, I was going to check his temperature. This grew to be very stressful, but no weight could weigh heavier than what was to come next.

Months after Kingston had his first seizure, he simply stopped eating all vegetables and meats. Shortly after that he stopped eating pasta and certain fruits. He was nearly four years old and wasn't speaking at the level he was supposed to. If he wanted something he would point to it, but without making a sound. I noticed that he would rock back and forth and walk on his tippy-toes a lot too.

February 4, 2015, I would get the worst news I have gotten in my entire life. I would be told by a developmental pediatrician that my baby Kingston was diagnosed with autism. Those seizures had been traumatic, but in this moment, I wasn't sure how I would maintain from that point on. I was crushed. It felt like a gigantic boulder was placed on my back to carry around forever. I mean, that is what the doctors tell you. They tell you that this diagnosis is forever.

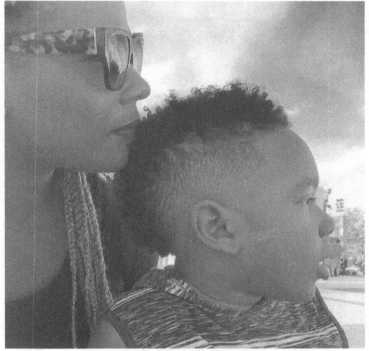
Disney Land with Kingston

Needless to say, I hit the ground running. I was determined to find all of the help that I could. I researched everything from therapies, to his diet, to state assistance, to a cure.

As I look back on it, I believe that I may have gone into a functional psychosis. I didn't take the time to deal with my emotions, because I was convinced that there was no time to be sad. I took all of the stress that was thrown my way and just harbored it in my body. No release whatsoever for myself. I was already going through a great deal of other transitions in my life that were challenging, not to mention the very simple task of trying to love yourself daily. At this point, Syleena didn't matter, only Kingston.

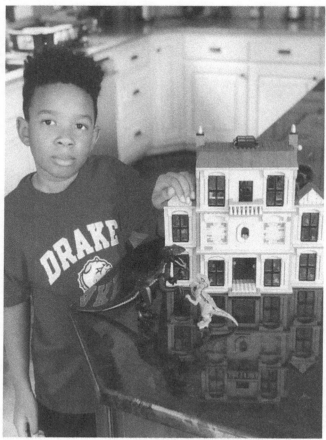

Kingston with his completed 1000-piece Jurassic World Lego set

I was so tunnel-visioned that I ignored the fact I had a husband and a son who got the same news, and that it impacted them just as much. I used to worry all the time about KJ having to defend and take up for his brother. I got pregnant again so that KJ could have a playmate.

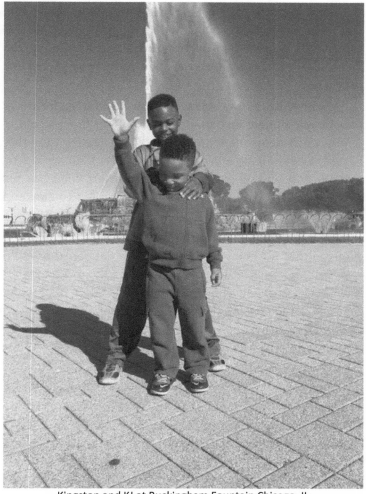

Kingston and KJ at Buckingham Fountain Chicago, IL

I wanted him and his brother to be best friends, since he didn't really have that in his oldest brother from Kiwane's previous marriage. How would he adjust? Would Kingston know what a best friend is? Would Kingston be able to play video games and communicate with him like a little brother should?

Then there is my husband. How does this make him feel? Is he okay? He has been through so much in his life and can handle a great deal of things, but would this be the straw that broke the camel's back for him? Does he feel like me?

I believe it was my straw. I hid my pain deep inside so that I could appear strong for Kingston and the rest of the family. I was determined to do whatever I needed to so that Kingston could have a great quality of life. I am optimistic that he will pull all the way through, even if he has his quirks. I just want him to be able to live his life as a man and have a real chance at life.

Oftentimes I have blamed myself for Kingston's disorder, thinking that if I knew why or how this happened I would feel better about it. Other times I am scared to death of what it could be like when Kingston becomes an adult, but I know that God is with us and there is a lesson and a blessing in all of this. Either way, this entire era in my life was the ultimate weight. This is the kind of weight that you can't lose. This type of weight, you have to learn to live with.

Meanwhile, I was gaining the weight that you actually can lose. I was finishing up my bachelor's degree in nutrition science, planning for a mini tour for *Chapter 6: Couples Therapy*, and trying my hardest to understand autism, when I realized that I had gained a quiet thirty pounds. What's worse is that I didn't gain it from eating myself to death. This weight gain came primarily from the stress of Kingston's diagnosis and all that came with it. I was so unhappy. When

I looked in the mirror, I had nothing but disdain for who I saw in that reflection. I was disgusted at myself. So many times I have lost the weight, and here I was again with it all gained right back.

Eventually, I got tired of being sick and tired and decided to use what I knew in conjunction with some new information and ideas from my nutrition mentors Julie Burns and Margaret Nicholson. The goal was not just to lose weight but to essentially figure out a plan to change my life. You see, I couldn't change the fact that Kingston was diagnosed with autism, but I could change my own diagnosis, which was deep sadness and unhappiness. My plan was to change this with diet and exercise. And with discipline, prayer, and positive surroundings, that is exactly what I did.

The Fighter

"Fight the Power" – Public Enemy

I was finishing up with the last leg of my tour for *Chapter 6: Couples Therapy* when I started to notice that my legs were swelling more often than usual. At first I thought it was from the excessive traveling I had been doing. I had flown from South Africa to Philadelphia. Then I flew from Philly to New York, and from there to Los Angeles. On top of that, I had driven in between those destinations to different cities to catch some smaller markets. So, it seemed safe to assume that my body had taken a beating with all this traveling I had been doing, evidently causing these symptoms, or so I thought.

When I finally got back to Georgia, I noticed that my hands were just as swollen as my legs. This was very unusual. My hands had never swollen like this before. Even though I wasn't really sure what was going on, I knew that this couldn't be good for my blood vessels. Through my studies at Kaplan, I learned that swelling can come from heart and blood vessel issues. I also learned that weight gain can contribute to this, and weight gain was something I definitely did. This was the year 2015, probably one of the most stressful years of my life. In February I found out that Kingston was diagnosed with autism. In June I graduated from Kaplan University, with honors, and in July I started the second leg of my tour, starting with South Africa. Needless to say, my stress levels had been pretty high basically the entire year.

Typically, I'm the type of person that eats pretty okay on the road, and I was dieting ferociously before I went on tour. I had actually lost about eighteen pounds before I went on tour. However, I didn't keep that exercising and eating regimen up like I should have. So, I got on the scale (which I absolutely hate to do). My eyes couldn't believe what they saw! It said a *whopping* 239 pounds! This was outrageous for me, when I generally try to stay anywhere between 175 and 180 pounds. At five ten, 175 is pretty thin for me, so I'm always closer to 200. I hadn't been that big since after I had Kingston.

Oh my God, I thought, *how did this much weight sneak up on me?*

Before I left to go on tour, I was about 210 pounds. This is still not ideal for me, but that would mean I had gained twenty-nine pounds in two months. This just seemed so unreal to me. With all of the knowledge I have in my brain, and all the dieting, training, athletic background, yo-yo dieting, and weight-loss counseling, I still managed to put myself at risk for not only heart disease, but also type 2 diabetes, not to mention the various other diseases that came with obesity.

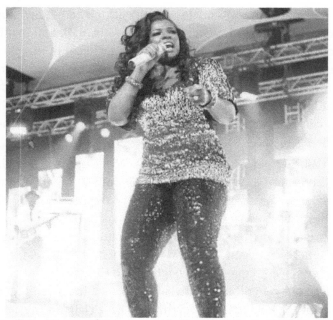

Headlining Women of Note concert in Bloemfontein, South Africa, 2015

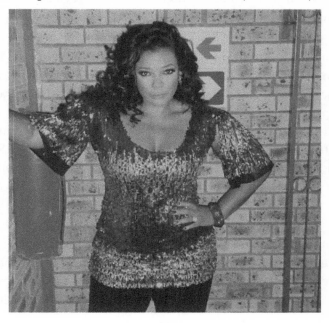

I decided to go to my family physician and get my blood work done to check my cholesterol levels, BMI, and insulin. Most family physicians don't really specialize in nutrition-based regimens. From what I was told by some of my professors, they only take certain classes in nutrition and that is all. However, there are some doctors, like mine, that actually study it and care about how it plays a role in their patient's health.

When I got my bloodwork results back, I learned that my cholesterol was a bit higher than normal at 187, but my insulin was within normal range. Technically, 187 for cholesterol is within normal range as well, but for me personally it was a bit high. My cholesterol is usually anywhere between 145 and 160. I felt that it would be higher since I had gained weight. Even though my numbers where okay, I still felt really sluggish, and the swelling was constant. I knew that something wasn't right in my body. My mood was also very irritable, and I felt very down more often than not.

I decided to call Julie, my nutrition mentor, and ask her about my condition. I started to explain some of the symptoms that I was experiencing, and immediately she knew what it was. She explained that it sounded like I was experiencing some symptoms that are a result of inflammation. She then referred me to a colleague of hers named Margaret Nicholson, who is a registered nurse. She told me that Margaret could give me some advice on a specific diet plan to investigate that could help me lose the weight quickly and safely.

I gave Margaret a call and explained my situation. Now, just because you know a lot about fitness and weight loss doesn't mean that you are not exempt from learning more and having a coach and mentor help you through your own fitness journey. Many of the trainers that I have had throughout the years have had trainers or have trained with someone to get to their goals. Margaret was empathetic to my situation. I talked to her about my diet and explained to her that my vices were red wine and cheese. I explained to her that I didn't drink the amount of water that I would ideally like to, but I wasn't a totally bad eater. She began to ask me questions about my lifestyle, not as it pertains to my workout regimen, but to my day-to-day schedule. She wanted to know how much sleep I was getting and how many times a day I was actually eating. As I explained to her my schedule and sleep patterns, I started to realize how stressful and inconsistent my life was. I began to see that my lifestyle inconsistencies were the real culprit to why I couldn't keep my weight off. Still, I just kept answering her questions as honestly as I could without hesitation. I knew that when I mentored people to lose weight in the past, I needed them to be honest so that I could create a plan that would be effective specifically for their lifestyle.

As a result of our conversation, Margaret was able to give me her professional opinion. She said she agreed with Julie and she felt that, because my lifestyle was so hectic and complicated, I was probably under an unusual amount of stress that contributed to the weight gain. Stress causes cortisol levels to increase, which can cause weight gain and inflammation. Inflammation in the body can cause water retention and swelling, which could be what I was experiencing. Furthermore, since fat cells are inflammatory, and I had gained a very quick thirty pounds, that would also justify her thoughts. Besides, research I came across during my studies at Kaplan University had revealed that sugar and dairy also contribute to inflammation. Clearly, cheese and wine were my vices, so I was pretty sure she was on the right track. In addition, I knew I had been under an extreme amount of stress. My job in itself puts high demands on me mentally, emotionally, and physically. Then there was Kingston's diagnosis that threw me into what I describe as a functioning depressive psychosis. God only knows what stressors were triggered during that time in my life.

The sneaky thing about stress is that it can be in full blossom, like those trees I talked about earlier, and you may not even realize it. It's a silent killer. Even now, I get scared when I think about the impact it could have on me. It's one thing to know that something is wrong with you, but it is a different beast when you are unaware of what could seriously hurt you. How can you fix something that you don't know is there?

Based on what I told Margaret, she decided it would be best if I followed a paleo-based diet regimen with a cleansing component. Basically, this means cutting out all dairy, grains, gluten, nuts, liquor, sauces, sugar, and adding certain lean cuts of organic meats, vegetables, certain fruits that are low in sugar, and herbal teas. She also encouraged me to drink half of my body weight, measured in ounces per pounds, of water daily. Since I weighed in at a whopping 239 pounds, that meant I had to drink roughly a gallon of water a day. That's tough to do, especially when you are a very busy person.

Nonetheless, I was fed up enough to do whatever was necessary to lose this weight. It wasn't about the way that I looked so much anymore. It was more about how bad inside I felt, and the fear that was attached to the hereditary predisposition of heart disease that runs in my family. After she gave me the plan, she sent me a box of safe homeopathic supplements to help with stress levels and metabolism, along with samples of protein shakes and authorized salad dressings that she felt could help me through my process.

I knew I had to have a certain mindset in order to be successful, so I created the twenty-one-day challenge that I now have available to everyone on my www.sheleanlife.com website. This challenge consists of a step-by-step program of directives that I would commit to every day for twenty-one days. The general premise of this challenge derives from the idea that it takes twenty-one days to break a habit. So, I figured preparing to win negates preparing to fail. In this instance, if I can give myself a solid start, I will have a better chance for a solid ending. I really just wanted to create a system that could keep me focused. I figured the way that I had been doing things in the past to lose weight wasn't effective long-term. Besides what I learned from Julie, I don't think I had mastered discipline within myself. I didn't want to start and stop again and again, because I knew that yo-yo dieting could also eventually lead to health problems.

On September 30, 2015, I started my twenty-one-day challenge and my diet plan regimen simultaneously. For some people it may be best to complete the challenge, then start your diet regimen, but for me it worked hand in hand. It kept me focused on something other than being hungry for the first couple of weeks. At the end of this book I have provided a 21-day journal for you to start your journey as well. Eventually the hunger subsided and the weight started to drop. I did a variation of workouts just so that I wouldn't get bored and cheat.

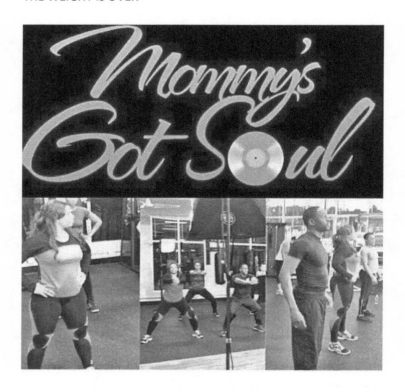

Of course, my main workout was my *Mommy's Got Soul* digital workout DVD that is also available now on my SheLean Life website. It's a full-body workout that needs no props so that you can do it anywhere and anytime. It's comprehensive, convenient, and effective.

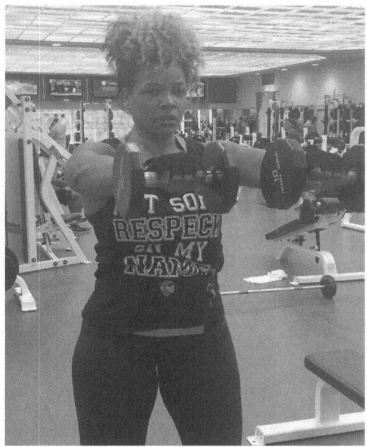
Strength training at Life Time Fitness

Other times I would do hot yoga or cardio with strength training at the gym. I had grown so fond of hot yoga that I eventually took the necessary steps and got my certification as a Yoga Alliance hot yoga instructor. In addition, I stayed consistent and ate clean. I prayed and meditated daily for strength, and as the months went by the pounds fell off. My focus and discipline were tested often, but God was with me. I felt strong, and I had already made up in my mind that I wasn't going to quit.

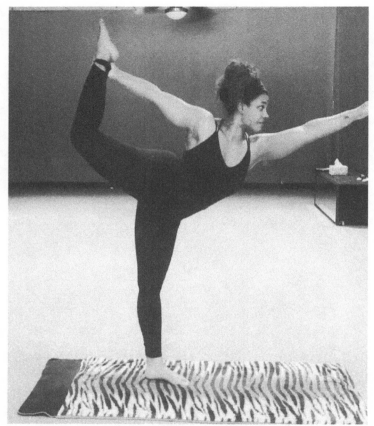

Standing Bow Pose at Hot Yoga of John's Creek Alpharetta, GA

Eight months later, I stood on the stage at the ATL Soulfest at 178 pounds, feeling confident and amazing in my skin. That was a sixty-one-pound drop over a steady eight months. I hadn't always been perfect with every single bite I ate throughout those eight months, but I stayed consistent with my workouts, and, more importantly, I kept a positive attitude.

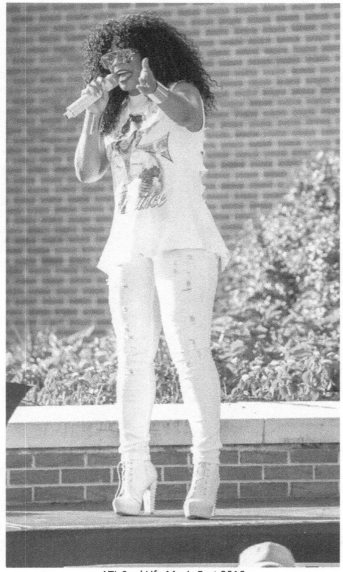

ATL Soul Life Music Fest 2016

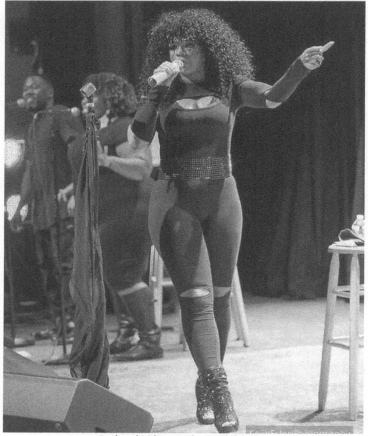

Bethesda Blues and Jazz Club 2016

You see, you can have all of the best intentions in the world, eat right, work out like a psycho, and still not lose a pound. Sometimes it is because you have hit a plateau and just need to keep focused until it breaks. I like to think of it as your body weight calibrating. Or, it could be that you really aren't eating enough or that you're working out the wrong way for your body type. There are many reasons why one cannot see the success one wants when following a weight-loss regimen.

I have learned that the number-one culprit for myself and most women that I talk to is stress. This is partly brought on by how you generally feel about your body and yourself. If you spend most of your day unhappy with what you see in the mirror from the moment you wake up in the morning, you could be accumulating unnecessary stress. You intensify this by putting yourself under ridiculous amounts of pressure to achieve a body goal that could possibly be unrealistic for your body type altogether. This is why I incorporated a lot of hot yoga into my workout regimen—to control my mindset and to ward off negative thinking. Hot yoga also helped me stay balanced hormonally, which in turn kept my anxiety down. It is ninety minutes of pure focus and determination in anywhere between 105- and 113-degree heat with 30 to 40 percent humidity. The hot yoga sequence is not only difficult to finish straight through, but it is done in front of mirrors so that you can see yourself and others make mistakes.

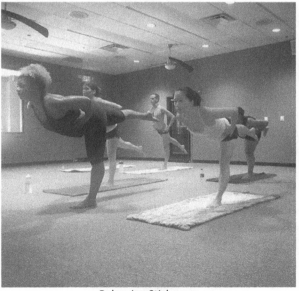

Balancing Stick pose

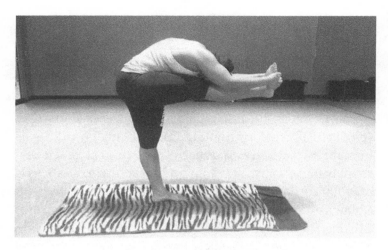

Standing Head to Knee pose

When I was training for my certification, we were taught that the purpose of this is to be able to see yourself and correct yourself while the instructor is giving detailed instruction for each pose. Essentially this is to ensure safety, which is a good instructor's number-one goal. While this is definitely a factor, I think that it also helps me see my true self. It shows me what my ego looks like, how well I recover from my mistakes, how well I take direction, and, most importantly, how long I will last. Being able to see all of this in myself allows me to be able to work on some of the characteristic traits in me that hold me back from my true purpose in life.

We all have greatness in us just waiting to come out, and you can usually reveal that greatness by challenging your discipline. Hot yoga challenges my discipline every single time I step foot on my mat to start a class. To stay focused, not sit down, give it 100 percent, and try every pose to the best of my ability for ninety minutes while staying true to the pose takes focus. But, more than that, it takes concentrated discipline.

I am a firm believer that when you willingly put yourself in a position to be challenged in a healthy way, you ultimately put yourself in a position to create change in your life for the better. Now, I have lost weight many times, and each time I have learned something new about myself, but this time would be a bit different. In the past, I learned how to train, how to eat, how much I needed to sleep, and the general theory of burning more calories than you take in.

This time I learned how to be okay with myself the entire time I was losing weight. Having this attitude and creating a peaceful mind would be the key ingredient for me to achieve my goals. I have learned so much more about how my mind works in relation to how I treat my body. I believe that I have mastered the ability to fight through diet humps, which really are just mental or emotional moments that will go away anyway. My relationship with food and my body can't be so extreme on either end of the spectrum. I have learned that I must create an environment that is synonymous to balance when it comes to my perspective of food and exercise.

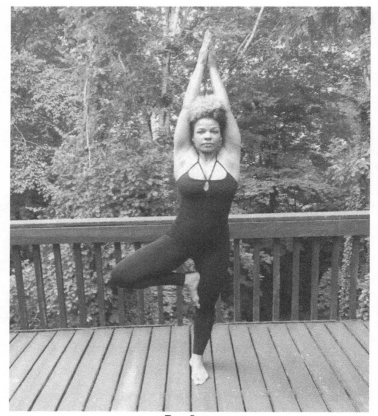

Tree Pose

Most of all, I must do what is necessary to minimize the stressors in my life. I love nutrition and fitness and it has been a huge part of my life, so I started going a bit deeper into it by achieving my certification as a nutritionist in addition to my degree and becoming a Yoga Alliance certified yoga instructor.

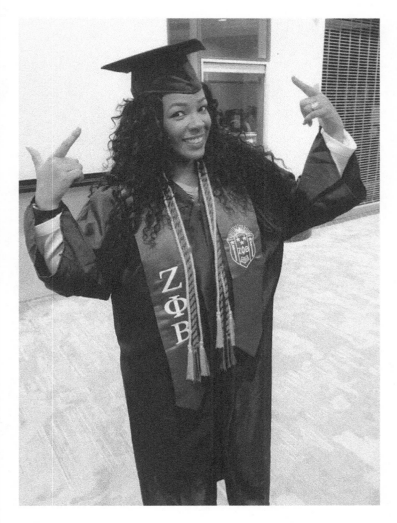

June 6, 2015 graduated from Kaplan University Summa Cum Laude with a
Bachelors in Nutrition Science

The Woman

"I'm Every Woman" – Chaka Khan

As I evolve as a woman, mother, singer, nutrition enthusiast, yoga instructor, and health advocate, I've become more focused on giving back to other women who have struggled with body image. I've been there, done that, and can understand how hard it is to get started with a fitness journey. Experience is the best teacher, and because I have experienced so much on this journey, I believe that I can inspire others to stay the course when it feels impossible to reach your goal. By now you have read about most of the woes that I have had with body image, and chances are you have identified with some, if not all of them.

Being raised in a family predominantly of women, I have realized that the conversations that women engage in have reoccurring themes about men, kids, and some form of weight management, weight loss, or diet plan. I know because I was not just listening to these conversations but engaging in them just the same. Because I have been through so many ups and downs with my diet plans, I have changed my perspective. What was once a singular issue that I had been trying to rectify from the inside out has now become a mission to help other women like me. This is the work that happens from the outside in. Helping others by doing the work on the outside feeds the love that you have for yourself on the inside. To encourage and create opportunities for other women to accomplish their weight loss goals and witness a renewed take on themselves reveals and fosters part of my purpose in life.

We are all here for service, and I believe that God has put me through so much to be able to empathize with others properly, and not just sell them a dream but to truly assist in changing lives. It is much like what I have already been doing through music. This time it would be through my passion for nutrition backed by years of trial and error and formal education. I believe that it starts with changing the conversations to focus on the healthy habits we develop and the products we embrace. It is about pushing each other to live healthier lifestyles every day and by being loving accountability partners.

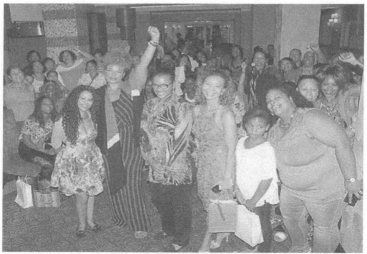

Eldorado Park Women's Conference

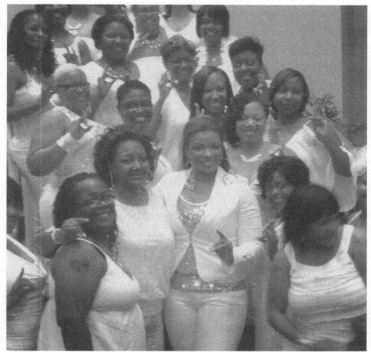

Illustrious women of Zeta Phi Beta Sorority Inc.

The question is, how do we get there and stay there? How do we teach ourselves to love ourselves enough to change bad habits? It's the same questions for everyone, whether you are single, a wife, a working mom, a stay-at-home mom, or a college student. Body image remains on the hot topic list. Our focus should be on healthy ways to maintain the body you want and celebrating who you are throughout the process.

To begin, woman have to take responsibility for their health. You can't be Superwoman when you have no energy. Proper understanding of nutrition is the key to building the body that exudes optimal health. Optimal health means not just physical appearance but building a body and mindset that can withstand sickness, stress, and conditional fitness.

Now don't get me wrong, we want to look just as good as we feel, but looks will fade. Your intention should be to have a healthy lifestyle that makes you feel good as opposed to just how it makes you look.

So I asked myself, how can I help women understand all of the different dynamics of a healthy lifestyle unless someone is sharing the message? Well, there is a lot of information out there about health and fitness that is at your disposal at any time, and most of it is great information and can help you reach your goals. However, I think that before anything, the word *lifestyle* must be the goal. We must change our thinking from "going on a diet" to starting a new lifestyle. This is how you set yourself up for lasting success.

The next thing that we must do to start on the right path is educate ourselves about our bodies. We must do the research, and I don't mean going on fad diets with friends and partaking in gimmicky cleanses to drop weight quickly. I mean truly figuring out where your body is by going to your family physician and getting bloodwork done. Once you get that done, go and see a dietitian and or a certified nutritionist and get a meal plan specific to your lifestyle and body type. Next, attain a personal trainer, or if you are a new mom or don't have the resources to afford a pricy gym membership and or a trainer, invest in workout DVDs or a digital workout that you can do anywhere. Of course, I suggest my *Mommy's Got Soul* digital workout and meal plan.

In addition, surround yourself with like-minded people who are into health and fitness and working toward that same goal. Most of us are as good as the company we keep, and we certainly can't accomplish any goals while we keep negative people around us. You don't need naysayers around you, constantly coaching you to fail. Make no mistake about it, there will be plenty of haters and dream stealers around you trying to get you to cheat and quit. Why? Because they are unhappy inside, and seeing someone who has been down in the dumps with them and who fights their way out makes them feel bad about why they are not doing the same.

When you decide to exercise discipline, there will be a lot of temptations to try and steer you away from your path. Ironically, these temptations will seem new, like they have never been there before, but the truth is they have become your norm and they only feel new because you have never challenged them. Like the temptation of eating ice cream daily alongside chocolate chip cookies while you talk on the phone with your negative friend about how fat you *both* are and how hard it is to change. This can become routine, like going to church on Sundays. Or how about how you have become used to having several cocktails after a long day, and trust me, I know what it means to have a glass or two of wine at night. When you have small children that run you to death all day, that may be your only refuge. However, too much of it can be the one thing that washes down the pill of guilt and disgust that you may already feel inside. Alcohol is a depressant and has a sneaky way of making you feel sorry for and about yourself. Or maybe it is social networking that happens after work at restaurants where everyone is freely ordering whatever they want to eat and drink and engaging in great, juicy conversation. In theory this is a great way to have fellowship and healthy interaction with friends and coworkers. You have literally convinced yourself that going out after work for happy hour is actually saving you money and contributing to your need to engage in grown-up conversation. Meanwhile, had you left work and invested those few dollars in a trainer or a gym membership, you would be benefiting much more. Or how about spending a one-time fee on an at-home workout program and meal plan and just go straight home after work. This actually could save you money.

Either way, the realization will come that what seemed to be simple things that made you happy have been the very temptations that have been holding you back, disguised as your normal everyday life. It will take time to get in a rhythm, but understand that it can and will be done when you work your discipline. It has been done time and time again by people all over the world, and you are no different. This is the motto that I live by. I have fallen many times, but knowing that greater men have fallen more times than me and still succeeded is the key to me staying self-motivated. Whether there are temptations or not, it will take roughly twenty-one days to break any habit.

I spoke about my twenty-one-day challenge in the previous chapter, and hopefully when you are done reading this book you will go to my website (www.sheleanlife.com) and follow it. I believe that it is part of the education portion of the journey that is necessary for long-term success, which is why it is free to everyone. One thing that is guaranteed to happen whenever you are on a path to becoming a healthier you and developing a better lifestyle is that you will fall and get up plenty of times. Luckily that twenty-one-day prep routine that I have created will always be there to help get you back on track.

Like I always say, even when we know a lot, we must always have something to reference back to. Even a trainer has a trainer. This is why I have formally educated myself on nutrition and fitness, because the personal benefits have been exponential for myself and for my family. Besides, I am surrounded by fitness and nutrition daily, living in the home with a retired professional basketball player and a miniature duplicate of him in my son. We are not just conscious about what we put in our bodies, but we are a basketball family.

Literally everyone that lives there plays or has played basketball. So, it is safe to say that we are a very active family. We are not perfect, but we definitely try to eat as healthy as we can, even with Kingston's issues with eating.

To this day he will not eat any vegetables other than carrots. He will eat certain fruits, but his diet consists mostly of chicken nuggets, pizza, pancakes, and turkey sausages. This drives me crazy, of course, but his doctor told me that he will probably grow out of this. She suggested a product called Juice Plus, which is a supplement that helps to fulfill the recommended dietary allowance (RDA) of fruits and vegetables required to maintain the proper nutrient intake that comes from these food groups. It comes in a gummy form as well as a powder that can be mixed with a liquid. My kids love it, and it helps to minimize the worries that I have from Kingston not consuming the proper amount of nutrients he needs for his immune system to stay strong. He is prone to febrile seizures that manifest from high fevers due to viruses and other seasonal illnesses. Therefore, I try very hard to keep his immune system as strong as possible. The safest and most effective way to do this, in my opinion, is through food. Since Kingston doesn't eat all of the foods that he needs to eat, I supplement his diet with Juice Plus, a liquid multivitamin called Calm, and vitamin D drops by Carlson.

Vitamins are a good way to supplement your diet and increase your energy. I am on the road a lot, which often compromises my immune system, so I take vitamins daily. Some health care professionals feel that supplemental vitamins are a waste of time. I've even heard some refer to them as "expensive urine," but I can definitely feel the difference between when I take them and when I don't. This is why it is important to seek advice from your family practitioner or a licensed dietitian. A certified nutritionist can advise you on a meal plan but cannot legally advise you on vitamin supplementation.

I believe that if you are a very busy or active person, chances are your body is frequently under stress. Stress compromises our immune systems. Certain minerals, like magnesium, and amino acids, like L-Theanine, have been known to help with relaxation or combatting stress and can be administered to our bodies through supplementation. However, it is truly a personal preference, and it is possible to get all the recommended nutrients that you need through a balanced diet. I just know that from experience I have not always had the most balanced diet, so whole food vitamins have been my saving grace. Overall, supplementation has also helped me to treat and balance my stressors and, in turn, stabilize my mood.

My passion for nutrition, health, and fitness has led me to become more active in the health and fitness market. The *Mommy's Got Soul* digital workout was the first product that I launched to lead the charge. Later, I added a meal plan and then created my SheLean Lifestyle website to house and administer those products. However, that is not the only reason I created the SheLean Lifestyle website. Actually, the website and vision had been established years before I even created the workout and meal plan.

Mommy's Got Soul was simply the key that started the engine. It started as a dream and vision that I created with one of my closest friends, Sheena Minard. I met Sheena while Kiwane was playing basketball in Italy. Her husband, Ricky Minard, played on the same team as Kiwane. We both had small children, with KJ being two months old, while she was pregnant with twin girls and chasing around a very active two-year-old boy. We were the only two American families on the team, and we lived right around the corner from each other. It was inevitable that we would bond, considering the fact that most everyone else only spoke Italian. So, essentially, all we had was each other. We weren't forced to like each other, but luckily we had similar stories and backgrounds.

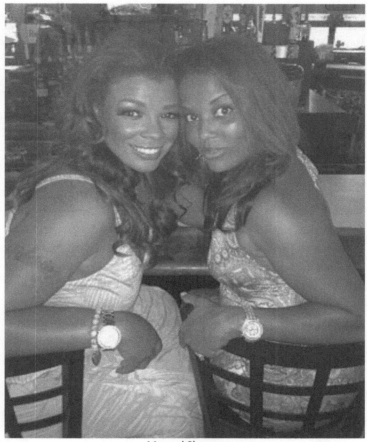

Me and Sheena

She played basketball and had a sister she was very close with as well as two brothers, and I played basketball and had two sisters that I was very close with as well as two half-sisters and a brother. Interestingly enough, we were what people today consider "basketball wives," in every sense of the word. Our lifestyles and family time spent together helped us build a bond that is still unbreakable today.

We frequently talked about how hard it was to maintain our health and our families, and we shared the same sentiments when it came to flying thousands of miles while being bombarded by baby bags and bottles. These stories and our experiences birthed the idea that would become SheLean Lifestyle, Health and Fitness company. "She" derives from the top of her name, and "Lean" derives from the last part of my name. We wanted to create an online company that would provide all of the answers to the many questions that we had as mothers that weren't immediately available to us.

Since we lived overseas in a country where English wasn't the common language, we found ourselves having to Google and research everything about motherhood, considering that we were new moms over there by ourselves, with no sitters or consistent help. I didn't trust anyone with my children who didn't understand what I was saying, so I just took KJ everywhere I went. Our mission was to provide a portal that housed information that would help educate and inspire all women of all races, ages, ethnicities, and economic status in the areas of health, fitness, motherhood, hair care, skin care, fashion, and anything else that we were generally interested in.

Most of all, we wanted to inspire and have something of our own. Not for just Sheena and me, but for all women. SheLean Lifestyle is a testament to every woman, and one of my heart's biggest desires is to see it grow, expand, and change lives through its services. When we returned to the States, we attained the LLC for the company, started searching for videographers for the first project, which was a workout DVD that later transitioned into the *Mommy's Got Soul* digital workout. As time progressed, Sheena had to part ways from the company and shift her focus onto some of her other passions. She went on to complete the courses to attain her real-estate license and later established the Minard Group with her husband, based in Charlotte, North Carolina. She is still very passionate about her health, and we constantly love to discover new and innovative ways to maximize our personal SheLean Lifestyles. We are still best buddies, with a relationship sealed by the bond of love and basketball.

Even though she has passed her energy along from our idea, I still have a burning passion to see this purpose through. My dream for SheLean Lifestyle is for it to become a household name and to grow into a food and supplement nutrition line, as well as a yoga-inspired fitness clothing line. I have implemented an ambassadors program to incorporate a broader mindset of the everyday woman and having them too be a part of the SheLean journey.

The ambassadors are a group of women who will go through a ninety-day fitness transformation, and, as a result of their successes, they will mentor and inspire a new group of women through the next ninety-day phase. We must be our sister's keeper. We must be that loving accountability partner. This is why we also highlight a woman of the month on the website, to showcase women who exude greatness in health and fitness and in their careers and personal life.

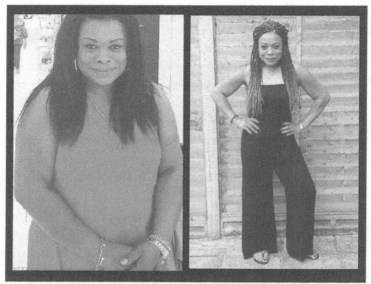

SheLean ambassador, Diane Bonner before and
after 70 pound weight loss.

SheLean Lifestyle is still a work in progress, but slow and steady wins the race. I want to make sure that this dream manifests into a lasting reality, a reality where women are learning, loving, and living their best life. After all, it is our health, our choices, and our lives at stake, and we must take control now. What we know and implement into our lifestyles as women will trickle down into our families in hopes to ultimately save the family.

Childhood obesity is on the rise, so whoever feeds the family breeds the problem. However, breeding is not the issue; bad eating and lifestyle is the problem. We must change the breeding ground. The woman is the source of creation. So, ladies, let's create a better world for our families to live in. If we are the initial nurturer and teacher of the child, then we can continue this God-given responsibility to our communities. You are every woman. Now look yourself in the mirror and say that three times.

The Conqueror

"Stonewall"– Syleena Johnson

I maintained steady breathing as I focused on the road ahead of me and the multiple colors, ballerina skirts, and hot pink socks worn by the other optimistic diva runners. Mile nine was the last mile marker I had seen, and my mind was feeling strong, even though my body was experiencing a fatigue that I had never experienced before. I was confident that my training had been adequate for this race, and I had run over nine miles in preparation for it. I followed the Hal Higdon half marathon training program in detail, but there were still certain things that you can't train for—certain things like anxiety, fear, and adrenaline, to name a few, and I had been experiencing them all at the same time, on top of my weary legs.

Nonetheless, I was not going to give up. I was determined to finish this race, whether it was on my feet, on my knees, or on a stretcher. I wanted to win, and winning for me was crossing the finish line, no matter what place I came in or how fast my speed was per mile. I had run plenty of 5K and 10K races, but I had never run a half marathon, and like anything else I set my mind to do, quitting is never an option.

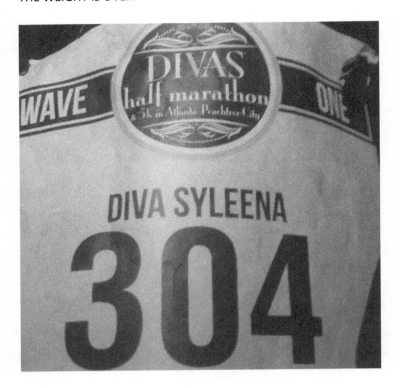

Keep breathing, Syleena, I whisper in my inside voice while sounds of Rihanna blast through my earbuds. I can tell that Eddy and Charita could really speed away and leave me if they wanted to, but they keep their pace right beside me. I must say, without them I am not sure how motivated I could have stayed up until this point. The very gesture to stay with me, when they could clearly be done with the entire race at this point, speaks volumes to their maturity and sisterhood. Women *can* work together, and this race was filled with women who all shared the same common goal, which was to finish. Women finishing for themselves in the name of girl power and to raise funds for iGoPINK breast cancer awareness charity. As I wipe the sweat from my forehead before it hits my eyes, I see faintly the next mile marker that would read mile ten. Butterflies started to swell in my stomach. Oh my God, I was only three miles from the finish line. Surely, I could run three more miles, I thought.

I kept my mind focused and my pace very steady. I was running at a pace of about ten minutes and thirty seconds per mile. This was a pretty good pace to keep up for ten straight miles as a novice half marathoner, and I started to feel pretty proud of myself, especially since my initial goal was to run at a steady pace of ten minutes per mile. However, I was a bit annoyed by the fact that I kept running into mini hills throughout the entire race.

You see, when you are running a long-distance race and you come up on a hill, you have to prepare your mind to stay calm. Running up a hill can take the absolute life out of you, because at that point you must use the muscles in your legs in a different way than you had been using them. It can slow you down a bit but accelerate your breathing, and if you do not remain calm and focused, you could trick yourself into believing that you will pass out! For me, running is mental.

I had already proven to myself that my body was capable of running for long periods of time by actually running at least ten of the 13.1 miles prior to this race, but in this moment, *believing* that I can run a half marathon will be the very thing that gets me across the finish line. Suddenly, Charita veers off and away from Eddy and me, and I immediately start to panic. *What is happening? Where is she going? Is she okay? Should we stop?*

Ironically, Eddy didn't flinch. She must have known something I didn't. I turned my head to see where Charita went because I couldn't hear her over the music that was playing through my iPod, and frankly I was too tired to pause it and ask Eddy. I saw her running toward a porta potty and felt a sigh of relief. I don't know what it would have meant for me if Charita had stopped the race, but I knew it wasn't something I wanted to happen.

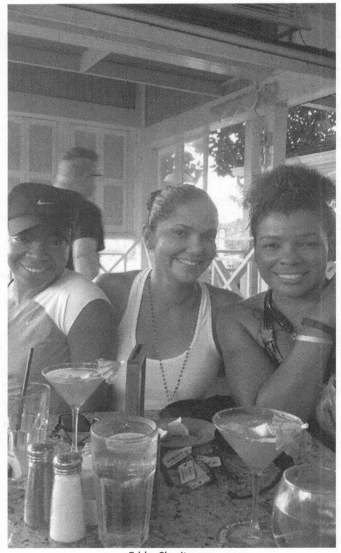

Eddy, Charita, me

I guess I really needed them there. Their excellence and experience in this pushed me to strive to be the same. They were older than me and more fit than me, and the calm approach they had toward the entire race from the beginning was truly inspiring. Charita is a real-estate agent, has two grown children, and has completed numerous marathons as well as triathlons. Eddy is a dentist and ran track in her younger days and has kept her fitness up all of these years by participating in these races and doing triathlons as well. To me, that made them real-life superwomen. It is hard enough being a working mother, but to find time to train for these races and still keep it together is just remarkable to me. I looked up to these women and still do. I aspire to be like them when I am their age. They have maintained their health no matter what, and you can tell just by looking at them. They were beautiful, and you couldn't find one wrinkle on their faces to tell their ages.

They were the ones who inspired me to run this race in the first place a year prior, when we ran the Hood to Coast race in Oregon together. That race was insane, to say the least. It was a two-day race where we split up two hundred miles between a twelve-woman team in a relay fashion, and it was nonstop. This meant we ran through the night, through sunrise and sunset. We slept in tents and vehicles and ate grain bars and recovery drinks in between. I was on a team of twelve black women who would become the first African-American, all-woman team to ever run the Hood to Coast race and finish. Forty-eight hours nonstop, and the great Donna Richardson was our team captain.

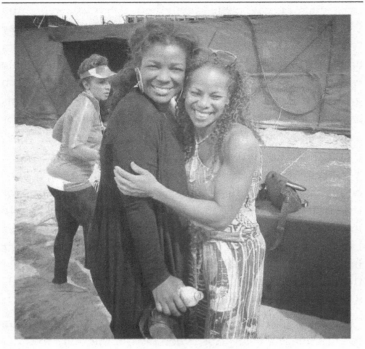

Me with Donna Richardson

As difficult as it was, the training for it ignited my love for running. It would be at this race that Eddy and Charita would convince me to run a half marathon.

I had an amazing experience with these eleven other women—all beautiful, all fighting for fitness, and all fighters. I learned a lot from them and will cherish those memories forever.

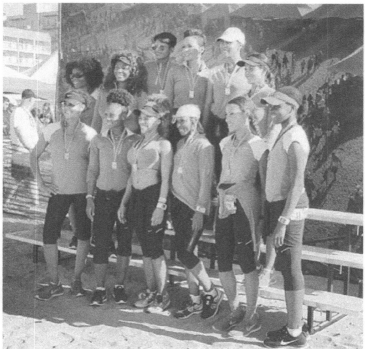

1st all African-American female team, Hood to Coast 2013

I just passed mile eleven and here comes a hill from hell. Lord Jesus, be a set of legs. My pace is getting slightly slower, and my breathing is starting to get a bit heavier. It's official— I'm tired as hell. Right before that realization started to set in, here comes Charita just as cheerful and energetic as at the start of the race. *Is she crazy?* I thought. *Who is this enthusiastic after eleven miles?*

Meanwhile, I'm starting to really feel it. Nonetheless, I was happy that I had both of them back. At this point, I feel like my spirit had already left and finished the race. I was just running as a shell. This hill was brutal. I began to get angry at the race coordinators. Why did they lie? Why, God? When I originally signed up for this race, it was advertised as mostly flat terrain. Well, I'm not sure what route they were talking about, because my eyes had seen me run at least ten mini hills and maybe three hefty ones, but if you let my body tell it, I had run at least three hundred hills. I was over it, but again, quitting was simply *not* an option. I mean, seriously, I had already run eleven and a half miles without stopping or walking, and I was determined to finish it with those same stats. There it was in the distance, mile marker twelve. Once I hit this marker I was pretty much a winner, I thought! Technically I had already accomplished a huge feat at mile eleven, since I hadn't run past ten miles in one setting in my entire life.

Breathing was getting harder, and my legs felt like lead as the anticipation and excitement was building, but then the unthinkable happened. I looked down for two seconds and *thump*! I fell to the ground! My God! I tripped over a huge crack in the ground right at the top of a mini hill. I swear, as I was falling, I could feel all of my hopes and dreams falling with me. I let go of every muscle I had. Charita and Eddy ran to my aid in despair as the other runners just kept going, I assume trying to stay focused. We were all too close to the finish line, and my catastrophic collapse just wasn't disastrous enough to stifle an entire race.

Honestly, I would have kept going as well. Yet it was still a fall for the ages. Hitting the ground wasn't enough apparently, God would have that crack be deep enough and that hill be slanted enough where I would actually tumble *and* roll. Consequently, I tore my brand new Nike running pants and skinned my knee and shin down to the white meat.

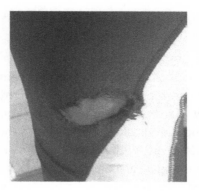

The pain was piercing, and the blood surfaced immediately, but my delirium made me jump up immediately and keep running.

I think it woke me up from a conscious slumber of tiredness that was coming. I think it was God saying, "HEY GIRL, GET MOVING!"

Eddy and Charita chuckled, and Charita asked me, "Syleena, are you okay?"

I just nodded yes, not having the energy to truly respond. We pass mile marker twelve, and now I am in a place mentally that wants nothing more but for this race to end. Pain screamed in my legs from fatigue, and blood dripped with every stride I forced. Here we go! My iPod was set to a 13.1-mile finish time, so the Nike app lady starts calling out kilometers.

I'm getting closer. Eddy and Charita run ahead, certain that they have done their part, but maybe understanding that I needed to cross this finish line alone. They were right. This race had now started to become synonymous to all of the races in my life. The start being the beginning of a test and the fall representing the part in your test that breaks you to your knees. Perhaps it represents the failed loves in my life, the disappointing moment when I departed from

Jive Records, the weight gain and the depression, or maybe the day Kingston was diagnosed with autism.

I have hit the ground many times in my life, but it has never been about the falls. It has always been about how I got up, who I became in those moments of my life, and how I finished. My Nike app blurts out, "Four hundred meters," and right before the finish line here comes the mother of all hills. Literally, the rest of the race was a hill! I realized that I wasn't just running a race anymore. I was running against fear, doubt, and depression, and running toward strength, hope, and faith.

"Hill, my ass," I muttered under my breath. It will take more than this hill to break me. It will be hard, it will be painful, and my body may not be willing to cooperate, but when you train the mind, the body will follow. My mind said *go*, but more than that, my heart did too. Two hundred meters and my legs are cramping, but I can see the pink arch with balloons and my husband and our friend Reggie cheering and videotaping the last steps. I see the many family members and friends of other women cheering and screaming with genuine happiness and support for their runner. Their eyes filled with pride as if they had run the race right alongside them, every step of the way.

I began to feel it. That wonderful rare feeling of accomplishment. That feeling of victory that stains your heart enough to be filed in your memories forever, right next to all of the other tremendous challenges you have conquered. "One hundred meters", she speaks over the music, and I can see the finish line plain and clear. Happiness overwhelms me as I push, push, *push*, like my firstborn son, except these were my legs! "Congratulations," my Nike app says, "you have accomplished your goal."

I did it! I reached my goal! I finished! I am a winner! I throw my arms up in the air! I see Eddy and Charita stretching and smiling as they intermittently drink the Gatorades that were provided at the end. Much to my surprise, there are half-naked musclemen holding our beautiful pink and black race medals and long-stem red roses. Now *that* was definitely a nice touch of gratitude for joining this race and fighting for a great cause.

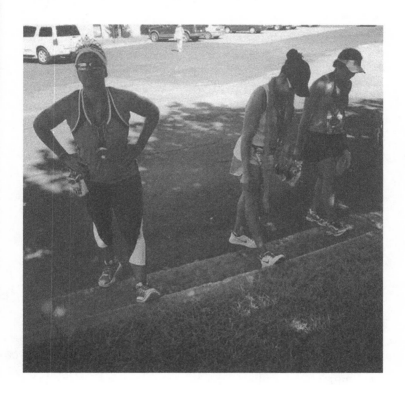

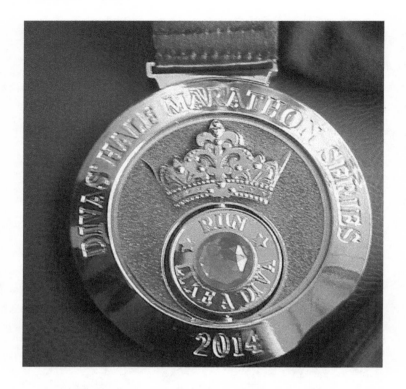

Shortly past them was a table full of champagne flutes, with each glass filled to the rim. *Nice!* Even though my feat was great, it's always the little things that tend to count the most. Someone truly put thought into how this race should end. Someone cared about the needs of a woman and really put thought into what would make us happy. That was a cool moment of realization, and even though I finished the race at the pace of a twelve-minute mile, I had run 13.1 miles straight, with no chaser, and I felt damn good about it. Through literal ups and downs represented by every hill, whether it was a big hill or a little one, I met them, ran them, and kept it moving to the next.

Now that I had crossed the finish line, the pressure was over. The anxiety was over. The Weight was over. Life is much like a marathon. There will be fears, there will be doubt, but there will also be bursts of bravery along the way. It's about having faith to the finish line, and the hills represent the many challenges that you will face.

You have to decide whether or not you will stay calm, control your breathing, and get over them. The only difference is that in life, when this race ends, it's over, so you had better do the work inside of that race so that you can finish and finish how *you* want. Who are you in this race? How will you evolve as this race proceeds? Those are the things that count. In the falls, during the hills, and in the moments of extreme fatigue—that is where you truly find yourself. That is where the true measure of who you are is revealed.

The truth is, the "Weight" will only be over if you train your mind to know that it is. If not, it will never truly be over for you, because stress, heartache, and the general pressures of the world will always exist. It is all about your perspective. The weight represents the stressors and pressures in life that we face daily, and you have to make the choice to stop letting it dictate your destiny.

Thankfully, I have learned that I need that weight in order to strengthen my muscles. And when I say muscles, I mean those mental muscles of resilience and focus that are needed to carry on in life. I have learned to use the weight to my advantage and change how I perceive and compartmentalize it. The weight is over when it comes to holding me back from accomplishing my goals! The weight is over when it comes to loving myself and accepting myself! The weight is *over* when it comes to allowing other people's perception of me to rule my mind and my spirit! I will no longer allow the weight to make me feel like I am not worthy of love and light. I will not let the weight push me into the corner of depression or weigh on my heart using guilt and disappointments of my past to create in me feelings of negativity and low self-esteem.

Instead, I will use that weight to remind me of how strong I am and how far I have come despite the weight. So here I am, looking in the mirror of reality, staring at the reflection of a mother, a CEO, a singer, a songwriter, an actress, a talk show host, a fitness and nutrition advocate and enthusiast, a yoga instructor, a wife, a friend, and now an author, and I'm okay with what I see. Standing underneath full-blown trees that have grown from seeds planted in childhood that once blocked my vision, now I use them as shade when I can't take the heat that this life can sometimes bring. I am still learning, and there are still more hills filled with lessons that I will have to learn in this lifetime. Only now I can say I am war-tested and love-infested. I got love for me now, even if no one else does. God is with me, and his tests have become my testimony. I have what I need to move forward, and when life knocks me out of shape, I will simply lift weights.

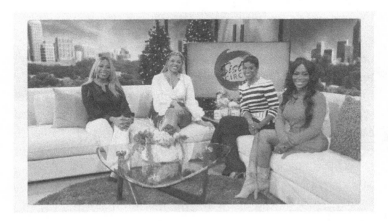

Sister Circle Live

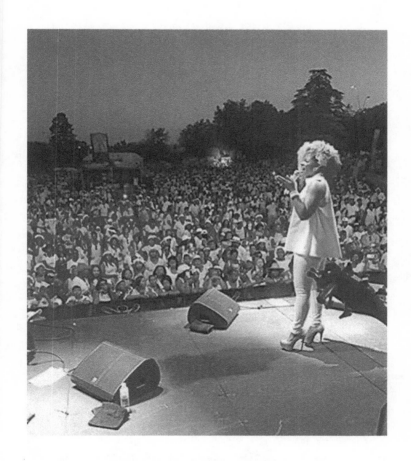

Headlining the Ebubeleni Music Festival 2016

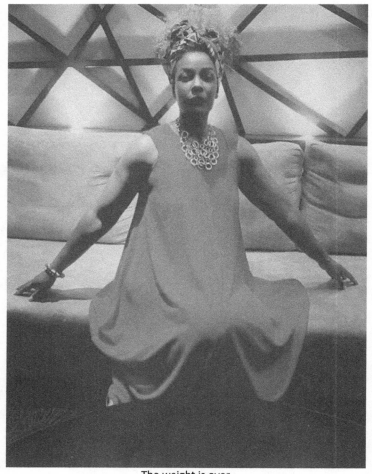

The weight is over

Syleena's Quick Tip Recap:

My Favorite Healthy Snacks

Eating the right healthy snacks can ward off hunger and keep up your energy in between meals. However, unhealthy snacking on chips, cookies, and cakes laden with sugars can actually rob you of your energy and cause inflammation in the body. Here are some of my favorite healthy snacks:

1. **Rice cakes**
2. **Green olives**
3. **Celery and hummus**
4. **Fruit**
5. **Almonds/nuts**
6. **Babybel low-fat cheese**
7. **Sliced avocado and sea salt**
8. **Hard-boiled eggs**

Syleena's Quick Tip Recap:

How to Repair Your Body after an Intense Workout

Today there are more avenues available that offer intense workouts in shorter periods of time. However you choose to get your workout in, remember repairing your body after a workout is as important as the actual workout. Preparation will assist with avoiding injury and increasing strength.

1. DRINK WATER

It's the simple solution that is the biggest pain for those of us who love juice, wine, and sodas. Benefits of water are unlimited and essential for proper hydration. Prolonged dehydration can lead to fatigue as well as all other sorts of disorders. Rule of thumb is to take your body weight number in pounds and drink half of that number in ounces of water daily.

2. STRETCH

A few minutes of stretching can make a world of difference before your workout and can help avoid a next-day leg cramp by stretching muscles after your workout. It's okay to stretch prior to strenuous exercise after a light warmup, but you will get the biggest bang for your buck when you stretch after the workout, when your body is good and warm. I encourage you to do some Yin yoga or gentle yoga once a week, just to ensure proper form and technique so that you don't cause injury. Many don't believe it, but out of all of the workouts that one can do, yoga is leading the charge when it comes to the most injuries a workout can cause. Crazy, right?

3. RECOVERY DRINK

Always consume some sort of recovery drink or a protein shake after a hard workout. Protein is essential for tissue repair and to rebuild muscles.

Syleena's Quick Tip Recap:
Don't Diet; Make it a Lifestyle!

I talk fad diets and unhealthy lifestyle in this book and how body image has been distorted in the mind since childhood. It truly comes down to this: don't diet; make it a lifestyle. Committing to a lifestyle change is the most important part to leading a healthy life. If it's how you live your life, then you don't need to make excuses for it.

1. Commit

Decide your health is more important than what others think of you. Once you are committed to being healthy, everything else will fall into place. Healthy does not mean skinny, and overweight according to national charts doesn't mean unhealthy. It's about your numbers according to your healthcare physician, how you feel, and your hip to waist ratio. Loving that version, whatever it may be, is the biggest commitment to yourself.

2. Find healthy ways to snack

Turns out an apple a day *can* keep the doctor away. Apples are high in fiber, which can help clean out the colon. You can add peanut butter to apples and other high-fiber fruits and grains to make it a well-rounded snack. Try experimenting with different healthy garnishes like guacamole and hummus on top of celery and raw broccoli stalks. Air-popped popcorn can soothe a carb craving with a little sea salt to taste, as well as a handful of roasted cashews lightly salted.

3. Use the benefits of healthy living to motivate the mind

Looking good and feeling good are just two of the many benefits that living a healthy lifestyle can provide. However, everything you do starts in the mind, so practicing mindfulness and meditation daily can help you to stay focused on your goals. Morning meditations and positive affirmations keep the spirit and mind in alignment with your attempts to maintain peace and happiness. Peace is a huge part of optimal health. We must fight for it.

Syleena's Quick Tip Recap:
Creating a Circle

Everything is more fun with help. Create a circle of friends or family that workout with you. Working out with someone else creates an environment for accountability. Give yourself that push by working out with a circle of friends. Most importantly, this circle must be clean in mind and spirit. It must be positive and encouraging. One bad apple can eventually spoil a bunch. The circle must serve as a coaching and cheering section all at the same time. By keeping the morale up, you can essentially keep the weight off!

1. Develop a sense of self-motivation

It's likely the moment your workout buddies have prior engagements or upcoming vacations, you too will miss the workouts. Therefore, always have a regimen set in place that can be done with or without workout partners. By failing to plan, you plan to fail. You will always be the most dependable person in your circle. Keep this in mind.

2. Change the routine

Don't just hit the gym or run on your street—change the scenery as much as you can to ensure the interest remains high. The key to staying fit is staying with something you love, so find a workout you love, and you'll stick with it. A repeat can sometimes cause a defeat. You can get bored with the same workout over and over again, then start to regret it and blame it for not getting you the results you wanted. Eventually you will convince yourself that all workouts are the same. I like to think of my workout like a love affair. If you find the one you love, you'll never leave it, and if you ever do, you will always come back to it.

How to Handle Setbacks

Setbacks can overwhelm the effort to be in the best shape of your life. Let's talk about how to make your setback be your setup for your comeback.

1. Start AGAIN, not OVER

Everyone will have a setback, be prepared to start again, not over. This means pick up where you left off like there was no time lost in between. If you constantly start over, eventually you will give up altogether. Focus on what to do better and identify what triggers your bad habits.

2. Every Setback is a Comeback

Give your comeback as much attention as your setback. Focusing on failure perpetuates more failure. Therefore, focus your energy on the comeback. The glass is always half full and never half empty. Visualize the finish line and not the race. Don't beat yourself up. We are all human and we are going to make mistakes. Victory is not measured by how many times you fall, but by how many times you get up and keep going. Anything is possible if you work hard. Persistence begets resistance.

Losing Baby Weight

Oh, trust me, I know! Been there, done that—twice. Here is how to get back on track to you!

1. Schedule workout time

When you are a mother, time is of the essence at all times. We have to plan and prepare to have an effective day. So, schedule your workout like you schedule feeding time for your babies. Treat it like a priority or it will become a chore. It should be as vital as brushing your teeth in the morning.

2. Mommy and Baby Workouts

Double the fun by incorporating baby time with your workout time. Put your bundle of joy in his/her stroller and go for a brisk two- to three-mile stroll up and down hill alongside a scenic route for the ultimate workout. Or, if your children are older, go on a family midday bike ride or rollerblade on the neighborhood trail. Places like Skyzone and trampoline parks are great for family exercise too. You can even track your activity with a Fitbit and get the whole family to join in on fun family step competitions.

3. Breastfeed your baby

Not only is breastfeeding the most cost-effective and convenient way to feed your little one, but it also contracts the abdominal muscles, helping to bring your stomach back to normal. Breastfeeding also burns calories and can lead to weight loss with a proper eating regimen. Plus, you don't even have to move when you do it. It also creates a bond of love between you and your baby, essentially making the baby feel safe and happy, and you feel like the great mother you are, knowing you are doing the best thing for your baby.

4. Be patient with yourself

Attitude is everything. Give yourself a break. It took you nine months to gain the baby weight, so give yourself at least nine months to get the baby weight off. Besides, stressing about getting back to your original weight is actually counterproductive, since we have now learned that stress causes cortisol levels to rise, which in turn causes weight gain.

Syleena's Quick Tip Recap:
My Favorite Workouts

Working out is something that I have done my whole life. It is pretty much second nature at this point. Even when I am not eating right, I still find time to get a workout in. It makes me feel complete. However, I stick to the workouts that I love so that I always want to do them. Here are some of my favorite workouts.

1. Mommy's Got Soul

When I am on the road I keep up my workouts with my *Mommy's Got Soul* digital workout. It's a sure way to get my heart rate up and get a total-body workout. The best part about this workout is that you don't need any props—you can do it anywhere, anytime.

2. Running

I like to change the view often for my runs. Everywhere I go I get a run in where I can. Whether it be a treadmill or a sidewalk near a hotel, the way that I feel after a three- to five-mile run can be equivalent to a long, hot bath at times. Not only do I run to stay in shape, but I love the constant pace of peace it brings. Running makes me feel strong. However, I don't run for long periods of time or on pavement much anymore, because over time running can be pretty hard on your joints, and we need to keep those healthy.

3. Hot Yoga

Hot yoga is my favorite thing to do. It encompasses cardio, strength training, meditation, and detoxification, all in one workout. It is probably one of the toughest ninety-minute workouts one can endure, but when it is all said and done, nothing can compare to the endorphin rush and the feeling of rejuvenation that it brings. It is the fountain of youth and the satisfying vice that I am proud to say I am addicted to.

Are you ready to take the challenge? Then go to www.sheleanlife.com and click on the 21 day challenge and get going! As a special gift to you, I have included a journal to help you keep track of your progress along the way! It's easy and fun and a great way to get a fresh new start.

21 Day Journal

Day 1

Make a Doctor's Appointment

Journal Your Journey

_____

_____

_____

_____

_____

_____

_____

_____

_____

_____

_____

_____

_____

_____

_____

_____

Day 2
Clean Out Your Pantry
Journal Your Journey

Day 3

Rid Yourself of Negative Energy

Journal Your Journey

_____

_____

_____

_____

_____

_____

_____

_____

_____

_____

_____

_____

_____

_____

_____

_____

_____

_____

_____

_____

_____

_____

_____

_____

_____

_____

_____

_____

_____

_____

_____

_____

Day 4

Get Your Mind Right

Journal Your Journey

Day 5
Create a Vision Board
Journal Your Journey

Day 6

Document Your Starting Point

Journal Your Journey

Day 7

Set a Goal

Journal Your Journey

_____

_____
_____
_____
_____
_____
_____
_____
_____
_____
_____
_____
_____
_____
_____
_____
_____
_____
_____
_____
_____
_____
_____
_____
_____
_____
_____
_____
_____
_____

Day 8

Get an Accountability Partner

Journal Your Journey

Day 9

Create a Budget

Journal Your Journey

Day 10
Plan for Your Hair
Journal Your Journey

Day 11
Buy Fresh
Journal Your Journey

_____

_____

_____

_____

_____

_____

_____

_____

_____

_____

_____

_____

_____

_____

_____

_____

_____

_____

_____

_____

_____

_____

_____

_____

_____

_____

_____

_____

Day 12

Become a Label Reader

Journal Your Journey

Day 13
Meal Prep
Journal Your Journey

_____

_____

_____

_____

_____

_____

_____

_____

_____

_____

_____

Day 14
Investigate Juicers and Blenders
Journal Your Journey

_____

_____

_____

_____

_____

_____

_____

_____

_____

_____

_____

Day 15

Drink Water

Journal Your Journey

_____

_____

_____

_____

_____

_____

_____

_____

_____

_____

_____

Day 16

Plan to Rest

Journal Your Journey

_____

_____

_____

_____

_____

_____

_____

_____

_____

_____

_____

Day 17
Set Aside Me Time
Journal Your Journey

_____
_____
_____
_____
_____
_____
_____
_____
_____
_____
_____
_____

Day 18
Create a Playlist
Journal Your Journey

_____
_____
_____
_____
_____
_____
_____
_____
_____
_____
_____
_____

Day 19

Buy a Journal

Journal Your Journey

_____

_____

_____

_____

_____

_____

_____

_____

_____

_____

_____

Day 20

Plan for Positive Social Activity

Journal Your Journey

_____

_____

_____

_____

_____

_____

_____

_____

_____

_____

_____

Day 21

Start a New Workout

Journal Your Journey

_____

_____

_____

_____

_____

_____

_____

_____

_____

_____

_____

_____

_____

Review Requested:
If you loved this book, would you please provide a review at
Amazon.com?
Thank You

CPSIA information can be obtained
at www.ICGtesting.com
Printed in the USA
FFHW02n1620161018
48815332-53013FF